D0843874

Stay Young
DETOX

JANE SCRIVNER

PIATKUS

Copyright © 2001 by Jane Scrivner

First published in 2001 by
Judy Piatkus (Publishers) Ltd
5 Windmill Street
London W1T 2AJ
e-mail: info@piatkus.co.uk

The moral right of the author has been asserted

A catalogue record for this book is available from the British Library

ISBN 0–7499–2212–5

Designed by Paul Saunders

Typeset by Action Publishing Technology Limited, Gloucester
Printed and bound in Great Britain by Mackays of Chatham Ltd

Contents

Introduction

The title *Stay Young Detox* is just that. If you are feeling good about yourself and good about your body, then now is the time to stay that way. If you are feeling that with just a little conscious effort you could feel better – fighting fit, energetic and fabulous – simply follow these programmes and success will be yours.

The Stay Young Detox is the key to a healthier and longer life; it is everyone's dream. The healthier we are, in mind, body and spirit, the younger we will look and the longer we are likely to live – within reason! If we have a zest for life then we buzz with energy and health. Staying young in mind, body and spirit is totally possible and really enjoyable. Detoxing for a healthier and longer life is here to stay.

Staying young involves a combination of mind, body and spirit, and you can embark on this programme when you are 25 just as effectively as when you are 65. Staying young is not about physical age; it is about the way you feel.

By maintaining your health you will have a better chance to look and feel healthy and young. If our bodies are fit and our minds willing we carry on to a ripe old age.

This is not to say that you can avoid illness completely just by eating healthily or keeping a positive frame of mind – but you will increase your chances and choices if you stay fit and healthy. Even if you know that your family has a history of a certain type of illness, at least you can take steps to reduce the effects or combat them for a while. There are foods to eat, treatments to have and exercises to do. Each of them is designed to give you youth and vitality. Optimum fitness allows you to do just about anything you want to, when you want to and how you want to – you have youth on your side.

But why detox? Why not just go on a diet and be healthy and get fit?

Detoxification is more than just diet and exercise. It is more than just adding more things to get you well. Detoxification looks at every aspect of your life and sees what is good and what is bad. To detoxify is to literally eliminate the poisonous substances – the toxins – from our lives. Poisons can be anything from downright life threatening to something that quite simply, taken over a long period of time, will interfere with our normal progress and stop us feeling good either in ourselves or about ourselves. The use of the word 'poison' is not a scare tactic either – here, it simply means stuff that our bodies or lives cannot use or do not need.

All levels of toxin are explored in this detox programme. The book is designed to let you find out what type of detox suits you best. It is individual and can be tailored to suit you and how you live now. The changes, additions or eliminations will not be the same for everyone, and the programme will not do the same thing for everyone; the phrase 'One man's meat is another man's poison', is very true. Some people are suited to a high-protein diet, while others get indigestion just thinking about it. A cheese board at the end of a meal could be what your dreams are made of, but it may be somebody else's key to an indigestion nightmare. We all need different things and detoxing to discover your own key to a healthier and longer life is what this book is all about.

Diet and fitness programmes are generally about adding things: adding exercise, looking at a balanced diet and adding that to your life, looking at being good to yourself and adding that. They can, however, miss out on the little things that need to be removed, or let some things slip through the net and continue to be less than helpful, or leave things that hold you up and prevent your progress. There seems little point in battling to feel fit through a rigorous exercise routine if all the time you are beaten by the need to simply cut out wheat from your diet to make you function well. Partner this elimination of wheat-based products with regular, healthy exercise and you will have sourced the root of the problem much more effectively and directly. You will feel fit and vital – a double whammy.

Detox leaves no stone unturned. It looks at all aspects of your life and takes away as well as adds to them; it gives you the bits you need, like, love and benefit from, and takes away the stuff that slows you down and gets you down. Detox is never just about food, and it is certainly never only about exercise. Believe me, exercise is my last resort – I know and understand the benefits but it doesn't make me enjoy the hard work any more. All I know is that I feel fantastic and virtuous when I am fit and toned, so it is my bargain with myself that the benefits outweigh the process.

Detoxing could actually show you that you need a hobby to pursue and make you grow – indeed, adding inspiration by removing boredom could be the only piece of the jigsaw missing. Adding something to your social or spiritual life, or to your general lifestyle, could be the overall outcome of your own detox mission, or it may make you take time to examine areas you haven't thought of before. Feeding your mind as well as your body can make you feel fabulous, and if you feel good, you radiate good. You simply cannot go wrong.

Detox is the true way to banish the bad and create the good, to give you health and a better life – inside and out. It is exciting and inspiring, and you may just learn something about yourself that you never knew. Staying young is physical, emotional and spiritual. Detox to stay young and feel fantastic forever.

WHAT IS BEING YOUNG?

To get to the heart of how to stay young, we need to look at what may make us feel old. Having identified these factors, we can eliminate or reduce them.

Feeling grotty, not feeling glamorous, not feeling attractive, being stuck in our ways, not feeling fit, feeling tired, feeling drained, feeling ill, feeling unappreciated. These are just some of the issues that you need to address.

Feeling young doesn't mean being childish or irresponsible or reliant on others. It doesn't mean all the awkwardness of adolescence and the hormonal changes of puberty. Hardly any of us would revisit those times of uncertainty and extremes. What staying young means is combining all the gifts that come with maturity and experience with the fun that comes with first experiences and youth.

We want to:

- Be healthy

- Be active

- Experience excitement

- Have energy to do what we want to do, when we want to do it

- Look good

- Look fresh and youthful

- Be flexible

- Be spontaneous

- Keep an open mind

- Be confident

- Be daring

- Have fun

- Throw care to the wind

The 9-pronged attack you are about to launch will ensure that every aspect of your life – both obvious and not so obvious – is looked at. All areas of your life will be uncovered, inspected and addressed – no stone will be left unturned. At the end of the programme you will have reached your goal of feeling young forever and staying that way.

You should attempt all 9 steps – you just need to decide in which order and whether they are all carried out at the same time or follow on from each other.

You should plan to complete all the steps at the same time in the same 18-day period. Allowing this amount of time will ensure that absolutely everything is addressed, so that after just 18 days you should be feeling approximately 18 years younger!

THE 9 STEPS

Your body

Step 1 The stay young detox food programme, *page 17*

The more I write, the more I read, the more I am totally convinced that each piece of food I place in my mouth makes a major contribution to my physical health. As long as I maintain a balanced diet – by which I mean balancing what we term as 'healthy food' with what we all love and know to be 'not so healthy food!' – then I am doing my body some good. There are some key foods that crop up time and time again. If you make these 'superfoods' the mainstay of your diet you will truly be feeding your body all the nutrients it needs to stay young, fit and healthy.

Step 2 The stay young detox looking fabulous programme, *page 36*

Looking great cannot be ignored. The boost that we get when someone says we look fabulous gives us bucket loads of confidence and generates a major feel-good factor. The programme will look at skin care, body care and treatments that will achieve major results. We will look at holistic treatments and indulgent but very necessary beauty treatments. Combining these two types of treatment will ensure that you look good from the inside and from the outside.

Step 3 The stay young detox total hydration plan, *page 65*

Water is one of the most important aspects of life. We are around 75 per cent water; our cells thrive in water and our brains positively come alive if truly hydrated.

We can go for weeks without food but take away our water and we would die in just days. If we don't drink, wash, bathe, shower, swim in or get treated by water, we miss one of the biggest tricks to staying young.

Water is crucial for detoxification. Detoxification is about cleansing, and purging and water is the best medium to use for this. It is natural and it is thankfully readily available.

Our skin is the biggest organ of the body. If our skin has the correct amount of water it stays elastic and fresh; if it dehydrates it becomes lined and tired. Our skin is responsible for huge amounts of water loss, but it also regulates our body temperature through water loss.

We will look at how much water we should be drinking each day and at how we can tell if we are getting enough water. We will look at ways to cleanse internally – as well as externally – with water. There are many different therapies that you can try, all based on water. Water has many different forms: heated, ice, steam, salt and fresh. Each of these forms, whether used singly or in combination, can be intensely therapeutic and extremely effective.

Immersing ourselves in water, surrounding ourselves with water or simply just looking at it, listening to it or smelling it is fabulously regenerative. The Stay Young Detox will look at every aspect of water in relation to youth and vitality.

Step 4 The stay young, stay fit detox, *page 78*

Exercise is one of the methods we can use to actually make us younger. A fitter and more healthy individual has a younger body and muscle structure than an unfit person. We can reduce the physical age of our bodies by taking up a safe exercise plan at any age. The Stay Young Detox will look at many ways to convince you to actually do some exercise!

Your mind

Step 5 The stay young indulgence programme, *page 83*

It is time to detox those thoughts that we should put everyone else before ourselves, and change them to the thought that we should fulfil ourselves in order to be able to have something worthwhile to give to others.

In fact, the indulgence step actively encourages you to break the rules and have that glass of wine that is forbidden in the eating programme and looking fabulous steps.

When we are young we tend to take everything for granted and expect that everything should happen just as we want it to. This doesn't leave room to see things that are special and to value them. Having time for ourselves in our busy lives or even just kicking back, putting our feet up and having a nice glass of red wine is essential. Total indulgence is incredibly good for the feel-good factor. Included in this programme is your absolute right to indulge yourself.

We don't look after number one nearly enough. Many people think that looking after themselves is selfish and self-centred. This is absolutely not true. If we only look after ourselves and ignore or actively neglect others it is negative and bad. If we look after number one in order to nourish and grow, we are much better placed to help others and have something to give. It is essential that we spend time making sure we have what we want so that we feel satisfied and good about ourselves.

Step 6 The stay young and stay in balance detox, *page 97*

Living your life in balance is possibly the biggest key to staying young and being able to do anything you want to do. You know what happens if the scales are out of balance – everything falls out of place. We need to pick things up and if possible mend them or, if they are badly damaged, throw them away. If the scales are in balance then nothing falls or slips, and nothing or no one gets hurt. Life in balance also means that you can try anything because it will always be balanced by something else. Yin and yang, black and white, male and female, dark and light, good and bad, fast and slow – everything has a balance.

Step 7 The stay young by thinking yourself young detox, *page 109*

In this section we will look at positive thinking, thinking yourself young, thinking yourself happy and thinking yourself well. Detoxing the negative thoughts and getting yourself into a positive frame of mind will enable you to do what you want in any situation or get what you want in your life.

Step 8 The growing young detox, *page 116*

Personal growth is the key. Growing young is possible. Discover what you believe you've missed out on and find ways to bring that into your life. Achieve something for yourself if you have spent your life supporting others. Take something out of your life to allow you to grow. This could give you extra energy to use just exactly how you want to.

Your soul

Step 9 The stay young, energised and spiritualised detox, *page 127*

Energy: what is it and how can we harness it? We use the term 'low on energy' and 'not feeling very energetic', but we simply mean how much we feel like getting up and doing something. In the Stay Young Detox we will visit all types of energy: energy flow, energy to burn, stagna-tion of energy, clearing bad energy and activating good energy. We will learn to feel our own energy, be aware of other's energy, and protect ourself from it or feed from it. We can control and grow our own energy, send it to other people, open it wide or close it down. We should be aware of it and act upon it; whatever we do we should not ignore it or be ignorant of it. It can be incredibly powerful and a life force of its very own.

Energise and spiritalise your life and see what has hidden meaning for you and what can give you vitality. It is time to give some thought to the more spiritual areas of your life. I don't mean religion necessarily but non-material aspects of your life that fulfil you – your beliefs, your energy, your aura, your very being. We can look at methods to develop these aspects and to explore them so that you can find a way to build confidence and support within yourself for yourself.

We'll explore a range of beliefs, therapies and approaches to find your fountain of eternal spiritual youth.

HOW TO USE THIS BOOK

- Read the whole programme through once from start to finish.

- Reread the steps that interest you most and decide what options you want to try first.

- Work out from your diary the best time to allocate 18 days to transformation.

- Photocopy the checklist (*see below*) 18 times.

- Collect or shop for essential foods and equipment.

- Get prepared for change.

- Commence!

The 18-day checklist

Every day

- Eat Stay Young Detox superfoods.

- Drink 1.5 litres (3 pints) of water.

- Do 30 minutes exercise.

- Do one step to 'looking fabulous'.

- Do one step to hydration.

- Do one indulgence.

- Do one empowerment.

Every other day

- Do one mind step.

SOME FURTHER THOUGHTS

What does staying young mean to you? If you feel that finding spiritual enlightenment will be your secret to eternal youth, start at the steps in the soul section and work back through the steps in the body and mind sections.

If looking great and feeling good are what give you confidence and energise you, so that you feel ready for just about anything life has to offer, start with the steps in the body section.

If you know when you have got things straight in your head about your own life and where you are in it and where you may want to be, start with the mind section.

If your muscles are fully flexed and your body honed, maybe it is time to look at the spiritual aspects of your life – how to use your inner powers and intuition to move forwards and how to trust your thoughts, wishes and desires. Wherever you start, your path will take you in the direction you need to follow.

Within each section of the programme there will be new things to look at, new ideas to consider and some things to actually, actively do.

Every journey starts with the first small step ... go on, take a big stride!

PART 1

Your Body

1

Food Programme

Following a detox eating programme (not a diet) will make you feel younger, more alert and more vital. It will put a spring in your step and add hours to your day.

The Stay Young Detox starts with food. It is about super nutrition and therefore superfoods. We all eat every day so it is the best place to start. As we adapt to our new-found energy levels and our bodies respond to the nutrition, it will become easier to slot in all other aspects of the programme.

The beauty of food is that we truly are what we eat. Once you experience the feeling you get when you eat healthily, it is very hard to go back to an unhealthy diet. When we see how fabulous we look just by changing what we put on our plate, then it makes perfect sense to carry on that way.

Feeling the difference makes the difference. The Stay Young Detox concentrates on some key 'superfoods', and then looks at ways to enhance them and make full meals with them. As I said at the beginning of the book, the more I research foods, the more the same foods crop up as fantastic for everything. The following plan lasts 18 days. Where it states that you actually must do something then you absolutely must do it; where it says that you can choose, you can be as flexible as you wish, but don't stray from the list of allowed foods.

The stay young food programme is part of the stay young jigsaw. It is part of the whole. Everything is equally important and nothing should be missed or ignored. Therefore read through the section, work out when is the best time to start the programme and then take yourself off to the supermarket and stock up.

One thing before we start. I will talk a lot about anti-oxidants. They are hugely useful and are believed to be able to reverse the ageing process to some extent. They protect us, and seem to be able to lower the incidence of major illnesses such as cancers and to delay the process of ageing within our bodies. This ensures that we can maintain optimum health with a low rate of deterioration and a high rate of regeneration, growth and healing.

This can be confusing, as we all know that we cannot survive without oxygen. So why do we need anti-oxidants? Oxygen is essential for breathing but when oxygen is involved in chemical change or cell activity in the body, it can be damaging and form free-oxidising radicals – more commonly called free radicals.

We can see this more obviously when we leave the cork out of a bottle of opened wine – it oxidises and goes off. If we scratch a car and leave the metal exposed to the air, it oxidises and rusts. Oxygen in this context speeds up the damage process. Making sure our diet is full of anti-oxidants that will destroy the free-oxidising radicals will slow down the damage process and therefore the ageing process.

Some substances speed up this oxidation or make it much easier to happen: pollution, car fumes, alcohol, caffeine, food additives, food preservatives, burnt food, too much sunlight and many more.

Diets and lifestyles high in oxidants involve living on fast foods, drinking lots of coffee and tea, living in a city and regularly drinking large amounts of alcohol. Any or all of these factors will lead to higher signs of serious illness and bad health, or to signs of premature ageing.

Diets and lifestyles high in antioxidants involve living on a balanced diet of fresh fruits and vegetables, drinking little or no caffeine, having a low intake of alcohol, and pursuing healthy outdoor activities involving getting plenty of fresh air and exercise. These lead to a fit, young body, a young outlook and a health status that belies your actual years.

I cannot stress quite how important antioxidants are in our lives. I cannot express how important it is to get these antioxidants from foods and liquids and not from supplements. Following a bad diet and just adding antioxidant supplements just doesn't cut it. Achieving a diet high in antioxidants does. The Stay Young Detox does it naturally and safely. There is no substitute for healthy eating.

THE 18 SUPERFOODS

1. Broccoli, normal or purple sprouting

2. Pulses, including beans and lentils, and seeds

3. Beetroot, fresh, boiled or pickled

4. Berries: blackcurrants, blackberries, cherries, cranberries

5. Cabbage: any type, red, green, or Brussels sprouts

6. Carrots

7. Citrus fruits: lemons, limes, grapefruit

8. Garlic, fresh cloves

9. Ginger, fresh root

10. Cheese, yoghurt and milk, either goat's or sheep's

11. Honey, any variety, set or runny

12. Nuts

13. Oily fish: any type, such as salmon, tuna, mackerel and sardines

14. Onions, any type

15. Rice: short-grain brown, wild rice, red rice

16. Oils: any vegetable, seed or nut

17. Tomatoes: any type

18. Watercress

You can also drink an unlimited amount of water and include any number of herbs and spices (but no salt) in your cooking.

These are the ultimate detoxification foods. Combined, they will give you everything you need to stay youthful and healthy. You should simply fill your cupboards or fridge with these foods and follow the programme for 18 days. You don't even have to think about buying anything else.

The way you cook and serve your foods can vary, as can your choice of foods. For instance, you can eat mackerel, instead of salmon with almonds, instead of walnuts served on a bed of rice, instead of lentils and onions. This small list of foods can provide you with infinite variations of choice. You will be amazed how tasty they are with very little thought invested.

Don't think: 'But can I have ...?' Keep to the 18 super-foods and see how creative you can be. Alternatively, if creation is not your bag, then see how easy it becomes to make your meal decision if you are limited to these categories. You will save hours in the supermarket and will only need to spend time on deciding which herb or spice you want to try for the first time. Discovering something new is no bad thing – look at the section on keeping your mind young. Do new things and feel fulfilled.

The Food Categories

Protein	Fruits & vegetables	Fats & sugars	Non-dairy	Starch
Oily fish	Broccoli	Nut oils	Goat's cheese	Short-grain brown rice
Nuts & seeds	Beetroot	Seed oils	Goat's milk	
Beans & pulses	Carrots	Vegetable oils	Goat's yoghurt	Wild rice
	Cabbage	Honey	Sheep's cheese	Red rice
	Onions		Sheep's milk	
	Watercress		Sheep's yoghurt	
	Tomatoes			
	Lemons			
	Limes			
	Blackberries			
	Blackcurrants			
	Cherries			
	Cranberries			
	Garlic			
	Ginger			
	Grapefruit			

The categories of protein foods, fruits and vegetables, fats and sugars, non-dairy and starchy foods have been included to make sure you achieve a totally balanced Stay Young Detox programme, which is very important.

Every meal should contain foods from at least two categories and some foods from each category should be consumed every day. You should not miss out a food category in any one day. This will ensure that you are eating enough in quantity and enough of all the right things.

Buy the food, open the fridge door, prepare a meal and tuck in. Feel the years peeling away.

WHY ARE THE SUPERFOODS SUPER?

Broccoli

The innocent green or purple broccoli flower is jam-packed full of goodness. It is high in antioxidants, vitamin C, vitamin E, vitamin B, calcium, folates, iron and zinc.

There is also a sulphur compound found in broccoli, cabbage and Brussels sprouts called glucosinolate that is reported to discourage cancer cells and lead to lower rates of cancer. This compound is released more efficiently when vitamin C is present, hence these vegetables should not be overcooked (overcooking results in the leaching out of vitamins from food). Broccoli may also lower the incidence of heart disease and stroke.

Beetroot

Beetroot is full of iron and all types of folic acid, which is needed for cell growth and foetal development, and helps to boost immunity. It is a liver cleanser and a kidney booster – a detox all-rounder. It is incredibly high in antioxidants. It helps to build the blood and cleanse it: just look at its colour – it's a vegetable totally suited to the job. It can help to regulate periods and menstrual cycles, and is bursting with A, B and C vitamins. It is also a good carbohydrate.

Carrot

This is another vegetable that detoxifies and cleanses. It contains beta-carotene: carotenes are the names of the bright colours of certain foods, such as red peppers, oranges and carrots. The beta variety is especially valuable for its antioxidant properties. It helps to promote good red blood cell production, which in turn is great for the circulation and for heart health. The beta-carotene in carrots may also reduce the risk of cancers such as bladder, cervical, colonic, prostate and breast cancer. It seems to be particularly effective against lung cancers, as beta-carotene can be converted to vitamin A, which builds resistance to lung disease.

Carrots may also help to lower blood cholesterol and are high in vitamins C and E. The old wives' tale that carrots can help you see in the dark is no joke, for they help to keep the eyes healthy, and also the skin.

Cabbage

Cabbage is high in antioxidants and may strengthen the immune system, lower the risk of cancer – particularly skin, colon and lung cancer – and it may lower the risk of heart disease. It is high in vitamins B and C.

Cabbage helps with digestion and colon health. It is full of folates and is therefore to be recommended if you are planning a pregnancy, as folic acid is essential for healthy red blood cell growth and growth of the developing foetus in the early stages of pregnancy.

Onions

Onions decrease the risk of heart disease and strokes and also act as an antibiotic. Eating a diet high in onions can increase the body's resistance to cancer. They are high in vitamin B.

Onions also help to prevent blood clotting during internal healing, and reduce cholesterol and decrease high blood pressure. They help to provide immunity against and to fight colds, coughs and bronchitis. They are also high in flavonoids, and may therefore lower the risk of cancers.

Watercress

Watercress is full of antioxidants, which reduce the risk of cancer and help the body to avoid or recover more quickly from infection. Watercress can help to prevent anaemia and is so high in calcium that it almost tops milk for content. It is also high in vitamins C and E, and in zinc, folates and iron. The nutritional value of watercress is heightened because it is eaten raw, so that no nutrients are lost through cooking. Watercress is purifying, stimulating to the digestion and increases circulation.

Tomatoes

Poor old tomatoes have long been eschewed by me when writing detox plans. This is because of their high acidity and their potential effect on the gut when you are making so many changes during a detox programme anyway. You simply do not need anything in the programme that might make you too acidic. However, the more I read and study, the more I have come to the conclusion that in moderation, tomatoes cannot do anything but enhance the body's health.

Tomatoes are major antioxidants, and they contain large amounts of vitamin C; taken together, these attributes may lower the risks of cancer, heart disease and cataracts. Tomatoes are high in flavonoids, which help to protect the body against cancer. Flavonoids are another form of antioxidant found in brightly coloured fruits and vegetables. They can be anti-inflammatory, anti-bacterial and anti-viral – very antioxidant indeed, so therefore anti-ageing. The most wonderful thing about tomatoes is that they are so versatile. Whatever you do to them you don't greatly reduce that goodness. Used in sauces, raw or roast, they are equally good.

Citrus fruits

Citrus fruits such as lemons, limes and grapefruits help to strengthen the body's natural defences. Lemon juice in particular is valuable as it is alkaline forming. It helps to settle any urinary infections and also to kick start the liver if it is drunk with hot water every morning. Wonderful for acid stomachs, lemon juice and hot water can balance out Ph in the body. Citrus fruits may reduce the incidence of cancers and lower blood cholesterol and improve the circulation. They are high in vitamin C, antioxidants, flavonoids, potassium and folates. They are also anti-inflammatory, and they reduce excess levels of sodium in the body and therefore regulate blood pressure.

Berries

Blueberries, bilberries, cranberries and other types of berry are incredibly high in antioxidants and full of flavonoids. They help the body to fight infection and are anti-inflammatory. They can help fight urinary-tract infections by preventing bacteria from taking hold of the bladder wall. Berries are high in vitamins B and C. Cranberries are also anti-fungal and may prevent the formation of kidney stones.

Garlic

Apart from banishing evil spirits and frightening off the devil, garlic is incredibly good for your health. Taking garlic helps to build the body's immunity and to fight infection, lowers the risk of heart disease, is great for the circulation and decreases the incidence of stomach cancers. Garlic is bactericidal, anti-viral and anti-fungal, and helps to promote a speedy recovery from colds, flu and fungal infections such as thrush. Garlic can also lower blood cholesterol, encourages vasodilation (increased blood flow), lowers blood pressure and lowers blood sugars.

Eating garlic fresh is preferable as no nutritional value is lost. Cooking decreases the value and odourless tablets have lost some of the goodness – however, they don't make your breath smell as much as fresh garlic does! With garlic as with anything – fresh is best.

Ginger

Ginger is a digestive. It helps with indigestion and settles and reduces excess gas (flatulence), which is no bad thing. It can reduce the risk of stroke or heart attack by preventing the formation of blood clots. It is also very warming and stimulating to the digestion.

Oily fish

The value of oily fish has been known for a long time. The omega-3 fatty acids found in fish can reduce the risk of heart disease, stroke and cancer. They can also lower high blood pressure, reduce the effect of rheumatoid arthritis and relieve joint pain, and are an anti-inflammatory and fabulous for the skin. Oily fish are also high in vitamin D, iodine and calcium.

Pulses and seeds

Full of calcium, folates, iron and potassium, small but highly nutritious pulses, which include beans and lentils, can lead to lower blood pressure and reduced blood cholesterol, and therefore reduced incidence of heart disease. They are rich in fibre, which is good for the gut and blood-sugar levels, as they travel more gradually through the digestive system than many other foods. This can also help with energy swings, evening out the highs and lows. The levels of iron and folic acids in pulses may help to fight anaemia and aid nerve and brain function, while the potassium in them regulates blood pressure.

Seeds are particularly high in zinc, and may help with bladder stones and prostate problems. They are a rich source of vitamins E and C, which may help to reduce the risk of cancer and cataracts. The linoleic acid in them decreases bad cholesterols, which in turn discourages blood clotting and the narrowing of arteries.

Non-dairy: goat's or sheep's products

Most people are slightly confused by the term 'non-dairy', but it is used to describe those 'dairy' products that have not undergone the same fermentation process that is used for cow's milk production. Sheep's and goat's products are fermented differently, which means that the final products are much easier to digest. They can help with digestive disorders and actually stimulate digestion. Many people have developed an intolerance or allergy to cow's milk products. They find, however, that they have no adverse reaction to either sheep's or goat's milk products.

Nuts

Nuts may be high in calories but they are also very high in nutrients, an excellent source of essential unsaturated fatty acids, and a rich source of potassium and fibre.

Nuts should be eaten raw and unsalted. They are valuable for their high levels of vitamin A, which helps to protect against heart disease. Some contain vitamin C and some have beta-carotene (*see page 23*), which can convert to vitamin A. This makes nuts high in antioxidant properties. They are also high in flavour and a good supply of energy.

Honey

Honey's a hidden secret. It can neutralise toxins, treat stomach ulcers, relieve gastric illness or upset, alleviate constipation, help to cure stomach ulcers and fight food poisoning, *E. coli* and salmonella. It can also bring down high blood pressure.

Honey is a very powerful bactericidal, and can regulate blood-sugar levels and balance energy levels. It can boost energy (and its consumption won't be followed by a slump in energy levels as happens with sugar), and help with muscle health. It is fabulous in small quantities for lining the stomach before drinking alcohol, and for helping recovery after a night of indulgence. It is also reported that if you take raw, fresh honey from your local area in small amounts it can actually build immunity against local pollen and reduce hayfever.

Honey is very acidic but benefits do come from really small amounts. It is also reputed to be a true brain food.

Oils

As is the case with nuts, there is a common belief that oil is bad for you because it is full of fats. However, the fats in oils are essential ones, so oils can be used without fear, provided this is done in moderation.

Oils are associated with the healthy Mediterranean diet, low heart disease and low blood pressure and cholesterol. They are full of vitamin E just as nuts are, and this antioxidant quality helps to keep them as the essential youth dew. Oils help to keep the skin moisturised and supple from within. They can help with joint problems as they oil the movement processes. Oils are also good for helping with efficient digestion and bowel movement. There are numerous types of natural vegetable or nut oil that can contribute to health because of their nutritional value, as well as adding flavour to your dishes. Don't be afraid of using fresh dressings containing oil any more.

Rice

Unrefined rice is a healthy alternative to any wheat-based carbohydrate. It can help to prevent heart disease and various cancers, and to regulate blood pressure. The fibre in rice can reduce the risk of colon cancer and bowel disease and keeps the gut healthy. Rice doesn't cause sharp rises in blood sugar, so it keeps energy levels continuous and blood sugar balanced.

Many people have intolerances to wheat or gluten, or even have allergies to them. Rice contains no gluten, so it is less likely to cause reactions such as bloating, water retention or anything commonly associated with wheat intolerance. Short-grain brown rice has a gentle scouring effect on the gut so it is very efficient in cleansing programmes.

Water

You should drink at least 2 litres (4 pints) of water in the summer or on warm days or days when you are active, and

1.5 litres (3 pints) in the winter or on days when you are resting or relaxing.

There is a whole section in the beauty steps starting on page 67 on the benefits of water, its nutritional value and its uses; whatever you do, make sure you drink the minimum every day. You will feel wonderfully recharged and your skin will be youthful and refreshed and fully hydrated even if you do only this.

Herbs and spices

Herbs and spices are hugely underrated. We tend to think of them as flavourings, something to garnish a dish, and to look and taste nice. However, herbs and spices have great nutritional qualities of their own and should be used not only to transform your meals into feasts, but also for the extra goodness they can add to your life.

Some common herbs are described below.

Chervil

This is full of flavonoids, which we know by now are great antioxidants. Chervil is cleansing, purifying; it helps digestive problems and it is a diuretic – so don't eat too much! Try finely chopped chervil with rice and goat's cheese.

Chicory

Full of flavour, chicory is another cleansing herb. It is a great liver tonic, and is therefore key to detox. Chicory is quite peppery and can be added to salads almost as a salad leaf for flavour.

Chives

Chives are again full of flavonoids, and are antibiotic and anti-fungal. They are commonly chopped and strewn on soups or salmon steaks – try both ways and taste the mild onion flavours.

Coriander/cilantro

Coriander is good for digestion, in that it combats indigestion. With its cleansing properties and refreshing flavour, this versatile herb can be partnered with just about anything – salads, soups, fish or cheeses. Open your mind and taste the difference.

Dandelion

Dandelion leaves are not just pretty flowers in the garden anymore, for they have now been recognised as highly nutritious. As a child, you may have been told that if you lick your hands after playing with dandelions it will make you want to go to the loo – well, dandelion is indeed a diuretic, cleansing herb. It is a great liver and kidney tonic and is full of vitamin E and iron. The leaves can be mixed in with salads, but go easy until you've grown accustomed to the taste.

Dill

This is famous with fish. You can try dill with salmon, or roast vegetables with dill sprinkled on just as they leave the oven. It is very cleansing and good for digestion.

Fennel

Balancing our hormones is the wonderful property of this tasty bulb, and the feathery leaves or seeds are also incredibly tasty. Try bronze fennel for a different look, and serve in salads or, again, on roast vegetables.

Marjoram

Marjoram is energising, antioxidant, anti-viral and cleansing, and is great for digestion. A strong flavour makes this herb highly appropriate for serving with oily fish such as mackerel.

Oregano

Anti-bacterial and anti-viral, oregano is full of flavour and its small leaves taste scrummy with Italian dishes. It's great with grilled tomatoes, goat's cheese and avocados – a detox *tricolore*.

Parsley

The best known of herbs, parsley either flat or curly is a wonderful antioxidant. It is also very cleansing and goes well with salads, fish and soups. Chew on the leaves and freshen garlic breath, or just to get the full nutritional value.

Rosemary

For many people the smell of rosemary still conjures up

the Sunday afternoon family meal. Rosemary is incredibly versatile and goes well with fish, salads and roast vegetables. (I can smell it now and am starting to feel a little peckish.) Rosemary is mood balancing, just as the essential oil of rosemary is. It is anti-inflammatory, stimulating and anti-bacterial.

Sage

Sage is perhaps one of the strongest herbs and is used for very many purposes, not the least cooking. It balances the female hormonal system, and is cleansing and protective. You can eat it or burn it to clear and cleanse. The Native Americans use it for blessings and in ceremonies, and it is the most widely used herb in space clearing (*see page 180*).

Tarragon

This is good for digestion, as well as being calming and sedative. It is great with fish and good with tomatoes.

Thyme

This wouldn't be a complete list without thyme. It is antiseptic, cleansing and protective. Chop the leaves very finely and add with coriander to brown rice; squeeze on some sunflower oil and lime juice – and you have instant fragrant rice like nothing you have ever tasted before.

To give you ideas and help, some recipes are provided at the back of the book (*see pages 187–203*). All are made totally of superfoods and they are truly delicious. The range of recipes will give you some indication of just how useful superfoods are for staying young, detoxed and totally cleansed.

Think about the flavours, the textures and the colours of food. In general, it is right to say that the more vibrant the colour and the more crunchier the texture, the more distinct the flavour and the more pure goodness you are getting. This does make sense because the more foods are cooked, the more goodness is lost and the more the colours fade and the soggier the foods become. Think of foods that have been left for a while – they go dull and lifeless and their colours fade. Foods that have been prepared fresh and served immediately, on the other hand, are bouncing with goodness, firm and tasty.

Staying young is reflected in what you eat – full of vibrant colour and energy or slightly wilted and fading. You can choose from this point on.

2

Looking Fabulous
Programme

There are few secrets about looking good – few, because although some of us actually know exactly how to look good, we don't have the time or motivation to bring this knowledge into practice.

GUIDELINES TO LOOKING GOOD:

- Eat a healthy diet rich in fruits, vegetables, grains and oily fish.

- Don't smoke.

- Moderate your alcohol intake.

- Protect your skin from UVA/UVB rays.

- Hydrate.

- Follow a skin-care/body-care programme.

- Keep your hairstyle updated.

- Keep your make-up updated.

- Use body treatments such as exfoliation, depilation and toning.

- Exercise regularly.

- Have a positive mind.

Looking good doesn't mean that we have to strive for a secret formula which makes us 'model-type material' because for most of us that is not a favourable image to pursue. Looking good means getting a glance of ourselves in a mirror or a shop window and seeing the person we are and want to be smiling right back and feeling pretty damned good about it. By including the above list in your weekly or monthly regime, you'll find that life will be great and you will look great and feel great, too.

The Stay Young Detox has pinpointed 9 points to looking fabulous. You should take these 9 steps every day during the 18-day programme. Where you are asked to give something up you should do so immediately. Where you are asked to start something you should do so as soon as possible and carry on every day from that point forwards.

9 Steps to Peel Back the Years

All the explanations for the 9 points are on the following pages; where relevant, the techniques that you should follow are at the back of the book (*see pages 204–218*).

Sun protection You must choose a moisturising product or sun-protection product for your face that has a minimum 15 sun-protection factor (SPF). This should be used every day from the first day of the 18-day programme for the rest of your life. Don't leave home without it.

Cleansing the toxins	You must give up smoking, caffeine and alcohol (except when you go for the indulgence steps!).
Beauty sleep	You should be in bed by 10.30 p.m. for at least 14 nights of the 18-day programme. You may read but must not watch television. Ideally, it should be lights out by 10.45 p.m. at the latest.
Dealing with cellulite	Every day, you should take a thermotherapy shower, dry skin brush and self massage.
Exfoliation	You should exfoliate every other day.
Moisturising	You should moisturise your whole body every day.
Depilation	You should remove unwanted hair once during the programme – more often if required, but a minimum of once.
New hairstyle	You should have your hair restyled and/or recoloured during the 18-day programme.
New make-up	You should have a make-up consultation at least once during the 18 days. Alternatively, you should clean out your make-up bag and invest in at least two new products of colours that are different from the colours you currently use.

You won't need to give up being human or to change your time allocation to fit in several hours at the salon or clinic every week. You just need to get clever with some parts of your 'care' programme, so that you will get gorgeous quickly. You'll find that a great weight will be taken off your mind. It really is that simple.

Looking good means feeling good. That can mean many, many things, but there is no doubt that an outward feeling of gorgeousness gives an inward feeling of gorgeousness and vice versa – so let's get gorgeous.

SOME MORE FACTS TO GET YOU LOOKING AND THINKING GREAT

Following a fabulously healthy diet packed full of super-foods will make you glow from within and without. Having a balanced diet full of nutrients and antioxidants will maintain the equilibrium within your body as far as fluid and Ph balance is concerned. We have looked at what types of food we should be eating and how we can use water as our very own youth dew, so now we can look at ways to take care of our bodies to look just fab.

There are many things we can do to look younger and, more importantly, to reverse the signs of ageing and to slow down the ageing process. Removing the elements that contribute to ageing from our daily lives will mean we look better for longer. The route to looking better for longer is to cut out anything that is damaging and put in all the extras that are beneficial.

The brilliant thing is that much of what we may feel makes us look older is totally reversible, or at the very least, can be much improved.

We can look at some of the things that affect our appearance and see just how simple it is to look younger sooner. I am not obsessed with looking younger, but most people would say that looking better would make them feel better, boost their confidence and make them feel that they could take on anything and win. Looking and feeling good is quite rightly pretty high up on our list of priorities. There are some things to consider before we actually look at the 9 points in themselves.

Amazing Skin

If someone says 'You look fantastic', it makes our day. Whatever has gone on before, it boosts the way we feel and gives us confidence to face the world with renewed vigour.

Following the Stay Young Detox will guarantee fabulous skin, a glowing complexion and a wrinkle-free smile – leaving just those lines that form when your grin is as broad as you feel good. It may just banish your cellulite into the bargain.

There are many routes to great skin but of course the most important one is the one from within. We have already looked at diet. The importance of a diet full of antioxidants, vitamins, minerals and nutrients cannot be emphasised enough. To grow and maintain wonderful skin, you have to feed and nourish it – the payback will be well worth all the effort.

Certainly, you can use various products on the skin of both your face and your body, but the most important factor is how you feed your skin. The 18 superfoods can do just this. They feed our skin with everything required to stay hydrated, plump, smooth, fresh, glowing and young. A diet full of antioxidants will almost guarantee that your skin and body will stay younger for longer. Think of the analogy of cars – if you don't take care of a car it gets old and falls apart.

It is essential that you see how beneficial and all-encompassing the Stay Young Detox eating programme is for the skin. I have listed here just some of the ingredients for good skin. As you can see, they are heavily featured in the Stay Young Detox eating programme, but just in case you need more convincing – here are some facts. Needless to say, all of the foods mentioned below are superfoods.

Nutrients for great skin

Selenium

Selenium works to produce glutathione, which is a power-ful antioxidant. It is detoxifying and protective. It is found in garlic, beans and lentils, onions and oily fish.

Vitamin A

Vitamin A comes in two forms, retinol and beta-carotene. It is reported to keep our cells and tissues healthy. As such it will also keep our hair, teeth, bones and skin healthy and in optimum condition. It can remove or reduce spots on the skin known as age spots – actually regressing the 'old' tell-tale signs in our skin. Vitamin A is not difficult to include in your diet because it is found in carrots, green vegetables and fish oils.

Vitamin C

Strong, healthy skin relies largely on vitamin C. We make collagen with vitamin C and collagen is responsible for keeping our skin plump and healthy. Vitamin C is found in green leafy vegetables, among which raw green vegetables are best. Citrus fruits, tomatoes and berries are also very high in vitamin C.

Vitamin D

We can produce vitamin D when our skin is exposed to the sun, but unfortunately, exposing our skin to the sun is not terribly good for us. We can therefore concentrate on eating the right foods to get this skin tonic. Oily fish, such as salmon, sardines, mackerel and tuna, is where you will find a high concentration of vitamin D.

Vitamin E

Vitamin E protects our skin. It can also slow down the ageing process of our cells, most importantly the skin cells. You will look younger for longer if your diet is rich in vitamin E. Some of the best sources of this vitamin are nuts and seeds, vegetable, sunflower and olive oils, and green vegetables, particularly broccoli.

Thiamine

Found in sunflower seeds, thiamine is important as a B vitamin as discussed above. It contributes to the growth of skin cells.

Zinc

This mineral is essential for good skin and the maintenance of great skin cells. Pumpkin seeds are a good source.

Calcium

Calcium is very important for helping skin cells to grow and develop. Great skin, nails, hair and teeth rely on good levels of calcium in our diets. A diet balanced in vitamin D is essential for full absorption of calcium. Green vegetables are high in calcium, as are salmon, watercress, sunflower seeds, walnuts and sardines.

Water

So, so, so important. Water keeps the skin plump, hydrated and cleansed because it removes wastes from the body. A lack of water leads to dehydration and dehydrated skin; and dehydrated skin becomes dry, wrinkly and pale. Putting creams on is no substitute for putting fluids in. Water is found in high concentrations in fruits, fruit juices and vegetables.

SOME FURTHER FACTS RELEVANT TO THE 9 POINTS

Sunbathing

Having a golden skin glowing with health does look good. Unfortunately, looking this good doesn't outweigh the damage and long-term ageing it causes. The importance of protecting our skin from the sun's harmful rays cannot be underestimated.

As we get older, our skin obviously ages too. If I said that 80 per cent of wrinkles, dehydration, spots and colour blotches are due to premature ageing and can be prevented and potentially reversed, then we can see that steps can be taken.

Tans come and go in the fashion stakes but they have never been in as far as skin care is concerned. We may think that a tan is just a warm glow for fair skin and a dark honey colour for olive skins, and that as long as we apply cream and then moisturise, the change in our skin is simply the time it takes for the colour to fade.

Well, unfortunately, this is just not the case. Sailors, farmers and builders, and indeed anyone who spends the day outside in the elements all year round, have thick leathery, darkened skin that reveals the rugged outdoor types they are. If we expose our own skin to the elements, the same effects will occur. Our skin will become dry, rugged and tough. Outdoor types are also outside all year round, so their skin builds resistance over a long period of time and can get used to the elements.

We, however, are very good at booking two weeks in the sun, then going out on day one and bathing in the sun right the way through our holiday. The fierce onslaught can only be totally damaging. Two weeks of a glow for several years of untold damage – not to mention the potential risk of skin cancers.

Unprotected skin will age faster, dry more quickly and become leather hard. It will have small, broken blood vessels near to the surface, and blotchy and irregular pigmentation, and will look a lot more tired than it is. Skin that has been out in the sun or exposed to the sun on a regular basis ages much more quickly than skin that is protected from the elements. We can't just blame holiday sunbathing; we should protect our skin from ageing every time we go outside. Winter, with its cold winds and bitter rain, can be equally detrimental.

The UVA, UVB and UVC rays are sent to us from the sun. Luckily the UVC rays don't get to us because of the protective ozone layer – these rays do the most damage. UVA and UVB do get to us and it is these rays that age and burn respectively. UVA rays will age the skin and lead to premature wrinkles, lines and spots. UVB rays are the burning rays and also the drying rays. It is also these rays that are believed to cause skin cancers.

We cannot avoid these rays because they are in every type of sunlight – in fact any kind of natural light, for even if we don't get sunny days we still get daylight and this can do the damage. It is important to make sure that your skin-care regime includes a protective moisturiser or cream with an SPF of at least 15.

Pollutants, alcohol and caffeine

Smoking and other pollutants

Smoking and pollutants in the general air have long been known as the culprits for premature ageing of the skin, not to mention the internal damage they do to our bodies. Car fumes, chemical products, computer screens, etc., all produce similar effects to smoking, but smoking is the most damaging as smokers normally have a much higher, more immediate contact with the pollutants in tobacco/cigarettes. A long-term, heavy smoker aged 45 may have the facial skin of a 65-year-old – it's that detrimental.

Scientists at the London School of Medicine have evidence to suggest that for every 10 years of smoking your skin will age by 14 years. It seems that the gene MMP-1, which is an enzyme that breaks down collagen, is much higher in concentration in smokers' skins than those of non-smokers. Collagen keeps our skin toned and fresh, so if we have less of it or if it is damaged then clearly we are going to look baggy and older. Not good.

If you think about it you can generally tell if someone smokes just by looking at them. Their skin looks grey or yellow. It seems to have less life and colour than that of non-smokers, and 'smoker's expression' lines help to give the game away. Wrinkles around the mouth show the movement made when inhaling, wrinkles around the eyes reveal the squeezing of the eyes to avoid the smoke. As a massage therapist I can tell a smoker from working on their body: the skin is pale and the circulation is not as good as that of a non-smoker; there is also a slight smell as the body expels toxins through the skin.

Smokers' skin will have more blackheads, less even skin colouration and be thinner than that of non-smokers. The skin will be less healthy as smokers produce more free radicals – the damaging waste products produced by the increased metabolism that comes with smoking. Damage from free radicals can be prevented if the diet contains large amounts of antioxidants: green vegetables, fruits, vitamins and minerals, etc. All of these 'healthy foods' are damaged or their absorption into the body is reduced if you are a smoker. The circle is incredibly vicious. If you smoke, it is best just to give up right now.

Alcohol and caffeine

We are all totally aware of how damaging alcohol can be in excess. Alcohol is a drug that can kill in excess, but in the right amounts, it can actually be beneficial. Red wine is packed with flavonoids that are antioxidant – they help the body to reverse damage caused by free radicals and can help to prevent the signs of ageing and to slow down the ageing process. Drinking the recommended maximum amounts of 14 units for women and 21 for men per week has long been understood to be safe.

Caffeine is less extreme but can also put strain on the body and help to deplete it of essential nutrients. It can 'speed' us up in an unnatural manner and make us dependent on the caffeine hit to function properly.

Alcohol and caffeine, as well as all the effects just mentioned, can make us look pretty grotty too. The cartoon picture of a large-nosed, jolly old drinker with a foaming tankard is an impression of how we could look if we drank to excess. The image of the coffee drinker sitting up late into the night with a bottle of whisky and cigarettes is an exaggeration. But both images are nearer to the truth than we think. The large red nose with broken blood vessels is a common sign of a heavy drinker, but bad circulation, pale skin, spots and small thread veins on the skin are almost certainly guaranteed if you regularly drink to excess. Caffeine will do the same, although without the vein problems.

Alcohol and caffeine are diuretic and will make your body lose essential fluid levels. Drinking too much of either will prevent the proper absorption of vitamins and minerals. Alcohol and coffee consumption really does not sound too good at all.

Beauty sleep

A good night's sleep is crucial for our health and restoration but also great for looking good. Bags under the eyes and a pale complexion can be banished with the right amount of sleep.

Obviously, there are situations and times in our lives when getting a good night's sleep is virtually impossible. Having a new baby, a big occasion, flying through time zones or dealing with emergencies are just some of the reasons why we don't get to bed at normal times. But for most of the time we can regulate our sleep patterns so that we get the most benefit.

Eating certain types of food will help you sleep, but there are other kinds of food that, if eaten too late in the evening, will keep you up and about long after lights out. Following a detox eating programme will keep your body functioning perfectly and this will always help with a good night's sleep. There are some other tips you can follow to munch your way to slumberland. Carbohydrates will help you snooze more soundly if you eat them 2 or 3 hours before going to bed. The old habits of drinking a glass of hot milk or sugary Horlicks shortly before you go to bed will also do the trick. A pasta dish if you are eating out or a round of toast dripping with butter and honey could also send you off to slumber. These are obviously not all superfoods, but there are substitutes in the programme. A nice cup of chamomile tea will relax you, rice can always be substituted for pasta, and honey added to warm goat's or sheep's milk will make a cosy step to deep sleep.

Drinking coffee late in the evening will make sleep fitful and broken, as will an evening on alcohol or, indeed, even just one drink. This is a difficult one because it is most common to have your glass of wine in the evening, or to have the traditional and inappropriately named 'nightcap' just before you go to bed. Smoking is also a stimulant that may prevent a good night's sleep.

Relaxing before bed is key. Dashing in from a late night or leaving a meeting at 10.00 p.m. and expecting to get a full night's sleep before a 6.00 a.m. start is almost certainly going to result in a bad night.

Take a hot bath. Drink a warm herbal tea. Use essential oils to relax. Listen to soothing music. Curl up with a good book. Write down anything that is on your mind so that you can clear your mind without worrying about forgetting anything important. Make love: the feel-good factor will send you off to slumber with a smile on your face.

Unfortunately as we get older we seem to find it more difficult to sleep. Just as children need routine, so do we in the sleep department. Going to bed at regular times and getting up at regular times will help the body adapt to the regular pattern.

The way we sleep is also important. A good, hard bed will support your back and help you stay comfortable during the night. The right level of bedding will stop you waking up because you are cold/hot/not covered/too smothered, etc. The right pillow will support your neck and help you stay comfortable. The right temperature in the room will also help to dictate how puffy your eyes are in the morning. If you have ever experienced a night in a hotel or a friend's house where the heating is too high or where you cannot regulate the air conditioning, you will have seen the effects next morning quite clearly staring back at you in the mirror: puffy eyes and bloated skin.

Sleeping on your back is said to protect against wrinkles because you don't 'smudge or crease' your skin. Putting pressure on one side of your face for approximately 8 hours a day is very likely to give you a lop-sided look. As we get older it seems that the skin loses its elasticity so the wrinkles stay for longer. We have all seen the old films featuring ladies sitting propped up in bed to sleep so that they can counterbalance just this problem!

Sleeping in a dark room will help ensure that you get a better quality of sleep – melatonin is produced in the body when we sleep. The darker the room the more the body believes we are in deep sleep, so the better the melatonin production. Melatonin is massively antioxidant and can combat free radicals. We need to facilitate the best production we can – so no more sun shining in first thing in the morning. Get some dark curtains and sleep yourself to good health.

Take the time to get the right bed, bedding and bed linens. We sleep for between 6 and 12 hours a day, so we should invest in the correct tools for the job.

Not getting enough sleep can cause stress, tiredness, an inability to perform at work and at home, irritability, and memory loss or slow memory function. It can also lead to illness as the body has lower immunity. When we sleep our body conducts major maintenance and production jobs: growth hormone is produced, and cell renewal in our body and especially the skin take place. We also process thoughts and emotions; 'sleep on it' is not an empty pacifier. After a good night of deep sleep we are refreshed and more alert, and equipped to deal with problems or situations, or to take up opportunities that seemed impossible the day before.

If you are tired all the time you need to take a look at what the causes are. If you are not going to bed until after midnight and getting up at 6.15 a.m. to get to work, then it is likely that you are not getting enough sleep, or not getting the right type of sleep that you need. We generally get tired at about 11.00 p.m., when our bodies are producing melatonin. If we put off going to bed much after this, then we are leaving it too late. Much before this and we will wake very early the next day.

A good night's sleep leaves you feeling fresh and revived, and ready to face the day looking bright eyed and brimming with energy. Put some work into getting a regular, full night's sleep and you will notice the difference almost immediately – depending on how much catching up you need to do!

Cellulite

Cellulite seems to worry some people an awful lot. However, it can be worked on and reduced or even banished. So no more worrying, just get working on it.

Cellulite can be due to many reasons. Most women in the West have some cellulite because of their lifestyles. Factors that contribute to it include the types of diet they have and how active they are, rather than their inherited genes. What, how and when they eat plays a big part.

Eastern and oriental women, who are raised with a different lifestyle and diet, are less prone to cellulite and are less aware of it. Some lucky cultures are less prone to it simply because body proportion and fat cell distribution varies from race to race.

Female hormones don't actually cause cellulite but they do contribute a lot to its formation. This helps to explain why cellulite is most likely to develop during puberty, pregnancy and the menopause, when the hormones are disrupted. In the same way, women who take hormone supplements such as the pill or hormone replacement therapy (HRT) are altering the body's normal state, which may increase bloating, or the body's ability to process fluids and lymph effectively and efficiently. That said, cellulite doesn't just disappear when hormonal shifts stop – unfortunately.

Our bodies always have the same number of fat cells. Hormones determine their size, distribution and accumulation. Stress, a sedentary lifestyle, posture, tight-fitting clothing and bad circulation, and a dieting/bingeing cycle can all contribute to its formation.

Men get cellulite – but their hormones programme it to collect above and around their waists. In women, female hormones programme cellulite to collect on the hips, buttocks and thighs. Cellulite looks different on men because their connective tissue is firmer and more tightly packed, and because their skin is thicker and has a higher percentage of muscle fibre – 40 to 45 per cent compared with 30 per cent in women. When the circulation becomes sluggish, fats and slow-moving fluid collect between these connective tissues, resulting in cellulite. The superficial appearance of cellulite can vary widely –

some people talk of the orange-peel effect and others just see lumpy flesh; sometimes the cellulite is barely traceable as the skin layers above are toned and healthy.

Regular exercise, a good diet balanced in potassium and sodium, correct fluid levels and good skin-care techniques can all reduce or reverse cellulite. Any product or treatment that stimulates lymph flow and manipulates flesh to aid detoxification and cleansing will speed up the process, as will the alternate use of hot and cold water, or thermotherapy, in any treatment or process. We need to get the body back into balance and then maintain this state permanently. The Stay Young Detox or, indeed, any thorough detox programme is really the only way to truly reduce or banish cellulite forever. A detox programme is about bringing balance back – so without even knowing it, if you are following the Stay Young Detox programme, one of the side effects is that you are reducing your cellulite. Not bad for a side effect. We need to look at the main culprits.

Bad eating habits

If you don't watch what you eat or even just grab something to eat without even considering the implications, and if you eat mainly prepacked foods or ready meals, it is likely that your diet is high in salt, fats and sugars. All of these ingredients are used to make foods taste more scrummy than they actually are. When fats, sugars and salts are broken down by the metabolism, much of the product is surplus to requirements – in short, there is very little nutrition left to benefit from. The main result is fat and sodium.

In women, salt, fats and sugars travel to the thighs and buttocks – traditionally a place useful for protection and to support childbirth. In the Western world, these characteristics are now surplus to requirements, but the legacy is big thighs and a wobbly bottom – nice.

Extra weight or rapid weight gain or loss puts strain on the skin cells and tissue. Constant yo yo movement will eventually result in sagging, drooping and stretched flesh. Lack of skin tone and elasticity results in our being able to see all too clearly what is going on quite naturally under the surface – our cellulite.

Dieting and not dieting

If you continually change the way you eat, eating plenty of food one week and practically nothing the next in order to balance the week before, your body will do everything to reduce the constant extremes of fluctuation. The body goes into starvation mode. In order to regulate the peaks and troughs the metabolism slows down in order not to burn fat. As a result, it has fat stores to call upon the next time we starve ourselves. The result is that even when dieting you don't lose weight because the body will not put itself in a position of jeopardy.

If you start to increase the quantities you eat over a short period of time the body will not be ready to deal with the overload. It will not be in a position to automatically raise its metabolic or processing rate, so you will feel bloated, your circulation and lymph system will be overstretched, and you will not be able to process waste and excess efficiently. This will result in the waste being stored in the body, mostly as cellulite, in the areas of the thighs and buttocks.

An imbalanced diet

If you eat an imbalanced diet you will not be providing your body with the essential nutrients required to process foods and maintain peak condition. A diet full of prepacked and ready-made foods is a diet full of colourings, flavourings, preservatives and sweeteners. It is also probably full of more sodium than potassium (*see below*). There is unlikely to be enough fibre in the diet and the fresh food content will be almost non-existent – not an antioxidant to be seen. When the body has been fuelled by sub-standard nutrients over an extended period of time the result is tiredness, lethargy, muscle aches and fatigue.

Sodium and potassium

A careful balance of sodium and potassium in the body is crucial to the efficient flow of oxygen, essential nutrients and waste to and from our cells. Sodium is found mainly inside the cells and potassium outside the cells. Essentially, the sodium/potassium balance within the body creates a fully functional pump – sodium absorbs fluids and potassium expels them. If the pump is out of balance due to a bad diet that is high in sodium, we absorb but don't expel or cleanse efficiently. Once sodium becomes dominant, movement between cells becomes sluggish, the removal of waste slows down leading to its build-up, fluid is retained and congestion occurs.

The short-term effects are bloating and fluid retention; the long-term ones are poor cell renewal and regeneration. This eventually causes irreversible damage to the internal structure of the cells. The Stay Young Detox will prevent this from happening because you will be following a healthy, balanced diet full of superfoods, and having a fully flowing supply of water in order to bring your cells back to peak condition.

All processed foods contain salts. We typically add salt when we cook and add more when the food reaches our plates. Our taste buds have been so underused that we need more salt than is necessary in order to get the most from any flavour left in the processed foods. Our taste buds also get used to salt, so that we need a little more each time we taste.

It is much easier to grab foods full of salt than it is to grab foods bursting with potassium.

Potassium is found in large quantities in fresh fruits and vegetables, and sprouted beans and seeds. Your diet needs to have twice as much potassium as sodium in order to create a healthy flow of nutrients and efficient expulsion of waste. There are various ways to get the balance right:

- Avoid processed foods.

- Never add salt when cooking, serving or eating.

- To get extra flavour in your food, add herbs, spices and garlic instead of salt.

- Drain any canned foods, especially fish, as these can be served in brine – which is just salted water. Choose foods served in oils or water instead.

- Check the ingredient listings on the foods you buy. Sodium, bicarbonate of soda, monosodium glutamate, sodium sulphite and sodium benzoate are all salt under different names.

- Increase your potassium-rich food intake. Eat more vegetables, such as carrots, broccoli, Brussels sprouts, cabbage and watercress.

- Increase your intake of seeds, and beans such as kidney, black and aduki beans.

- Eat raw vegetables for their raw goodness. If raw vegetables are not to your taste, lightly grill, shallow fry, roast or stir fry them. Keep the goodness in the food not in the pan.

Intolerances

Personal food intolerances, if not addressed, can result in a build-up of substances that the body finds difficult to process. If your body is dealing with a food it cannot digest or assimilate it won't be processing or eliminating efficiently. Fluid retention and bloating will increase the appearance of cellulite. Many people have an intolerance to some very common foods, ranging from simply feeling bloated after eating them to feeling sleepy, drugged or actually quite ill. We are not looking at actual allergies either – just foods that our bodies simply don't get on with. Foods that often cause such signs include:

- Dairy products
- Caffeine
- Alcohol
- Malt
- Yeast

- Wheat-based products
- Barley
- Maize
- Rye
- Refined flours
- Chocolate
- Refined sugar
- Refined starch

The easiest way to detect an intolerance is to identify what you depend on in your diet or what you tend to crave on a regular basis. The foods you eat a lot of and regularly, such as bread or cheese, could be doing more harm than good and may need to be reduced or eliminated from your diet. If your body doesn't get on with them, don't spend time with them! Once they are eliminated your body can get back into balance more easily.

Posture

Standing up straight does a world of good for our self-image. We stoop or lean forwards or have rounded shoulders for many reasons. We suffer from bad backs due to incorrect posture, and poor feet due to bad walking habits.

Our bodies are designed with sufficient space inside for our internal organs and systems to function correctly without hindrance. Changing this space through bad posture results in the body having to operate in an unnatural and forced environment. Restricted blood flow, an inability to breathe deeply, squashed flesh, constricted stomach movement and muscle shortening cause an inefficient flow of blood, lymph and waste within the body. The result is congestion, which leads to cellulite.

Tight fits

Another way in which we destroy the spacing in our bodies is by wearing restrictive or tight clothing. I remember working in a clothes shop as a Saturday girl and actually having a coat hanger on standby for use by clients when trying to do up the zip on impossibly tight jeans. I also remember wide belts that wedged themselves rather attractively in the space between the bust and hips, for a svelte and fashionable look. This may have been before or after your particular fashion era, but whatever the timing, there is always a trend to look thinner than we actually are. All these fashions restrict not only normal day-to-day comfort and practicality, but also, more importantly, natural movement within the body. This restriction results in congestion and so increases the likelihood of cellulite.

Inactivity

One of the main systems for processing waste in our bodies is called the lymph system. It doesn't have a pump or an automatic action, but relies entirely upon our muscle movement and on gravity to work. If we sit still and don't move our muscles, the lymph system doesn't get to process as efficiently as it can when we are active. This can result in stagnation or pooling of waste.

In any one day we typically spend 8 hours lying down and 8 hours sitting down. The remainder is split between standing and walking. We lie down to sleep, sit in a car, on the bus, on the train, at a desk, when watching a movie or in front of the television; we sit down to eat (mostly), stand when talking to colleagues or neighbours, sit with young children while they are going to sleep and sit down and put our feet up for a rest.

We know that mobility is important in elderly or ill people because it prevents muscle wastage, bed sores, weakness, oedema, bad circulation and poor respiration, but we never stop to think that any of these effects might happen to us through lack of movement. However, if we don't take care our ankles can become bloated or our circulation sluggish just through our normal, day-to-day existence.

Take a look at your daily activity levels. How much do you sit down? How often do you take the car when you can walk instead? How often does your leisure activity include sitting or standing still? Change just one of these each day and you will notice the effects on your circulation almost immediately. Good circulation means efficient processing and elimination of waste, which in turn eliminates cellulite.

There are many ways to stimulate lymph flow:

- Exercise

- Any kind of movement

- Alternate use of hot and cold temperatures (thermotherapy)

- Self massage

- Dry skin brushing

Doing some form of exercise for 30 minutes every day of the 18-day Stay Young Detox programme will help immensely. It will improve your muscle tone, which will improve the appearance of your flesh, and it will increase circulation and lymph flow. This in turn will improve elimination of waste and keep your body toned, glowing and in tip-top condition – the glow of youth can be achieved with just a few small changes.

Body treatments

Looking after our skin from within is the most important step we can take to make sure our skin is healthy. It means that the cells are developing wonderfully healthily right from the start. Cleaning and hydrating the skin from the outside makes the new skin shine through. The light reflects much more healthily from new, plump cells than it does from older, staler cells.

There seems little point in having wonderful skin if you cannot see it for the older, dead cells hovering around on the surface. Dry skin brushing, exfoliation and self massage are key to banishing cellulite. The instructions for these are at the back of the book (*see pages 207–211*). Follow them daily and notice how your skin becomes taut and toned.

Exfoliation, moisturising and depilation

These treatments are fairly self explanatory. Exfoliation (*see also page 211*) sloughs off dead skin cells so that your newer, younger self can shine through and make you glow with youth.

Moisturising (*see also page 62*) protects the surface of the skin's layers, and enhances the look of the skin so that it reflects back the light, making us look wonderful.

Depilation, whether by waxing, using a hair-removal cream, shaving or even permanent removal by laser, makes us feel trimmed and neat and ready for any short-notice call to the pool or an unexpected summer's day out.

Being prepared and maintained makes us feel ready for just about anything. Doing things on the spur of the moment is exciting and exhilarating – what a flash of youth!

Hairstyles and make-up

This is where we can get really girly. Whenever we face a life change, a crisis, a new relationship, a new job or just about anything monumental, what do we do? We get a haircut.

This is something that we can do to make a physical change. It can happen within an hour or so and it can make us look completely different, like new, younger, more sassy, more confident, softer, and more intelligent – just about anything we want really.

The so-called 'image makers' use hairstyles to tell a whole new story. The same goes for cosmetics. Changing from a pink-based lip colour to an orange-based one can result in a total transformation for the better or a total disaster. Softening the eyes with a pastel shadow as opposed to a thick black line of kohl can provide a whole new look in seconds.

Now I am not suggesting that we all sign up for a make-over (although it would be rather fabulous to see what they would make of what they were presented with, wouldn't it!). What I am suggesting is that we should try our own personal make-overs on a fairly regular basis. A change is as good as a rest and it may just give you a total new outlook on yourself.

Update and modernise is the key. I don't mean doing something different just for the sake of it, but I do mean trying something different that could make you feel a whole lot different.

Take yourself off to the hairdresser; if you are not confident that your current stylist can handle the job ask a friend whose hair you think looks good and is cut well to provide a recommendation. Show the hairdresser lots of pictures and ideas of what you want and don't lose all sense of speech when you are asked 'So, what are we doing today?' Be sure to practise what you want to say and then don't back down.

You may still have the same hairstyle that you left school with – it needs updating. You may have a style that was easy to care for when you had the children; as they are now at university you could probably afford a bit more time to spend on your hair – get a change. You may have settled for a style that denotes that you are getting a bit older – well, update; we are not talking mutton dressed as lamb, but we are talking a style that makes you look your best, rather than something you are getting by with or putting up with.

You may never have considered colouring your hair because long ago doing so (or perming your hair) could have been a disaster. Techniques and products are so much more sophisticated these days that any colour or treatment usually looks absolutely fabulous, lasts a good time longer and then fades or grows out quite naturally.

If ever we go out to a do or function or with friends we always wash our hair to look good. Why not have a new style and colour and look just fabulous? Hair grows and it is totally renewable, so experiment and have some fun.

It is exactly the same with cosmetics. There are so many brands around that there is almost too much choice, but it is likely that we have the same make-up routine that we established 10 years ago. We probably don't change the make-up we wear between daytime and evening – just put more on. The Stay Young Detox will require that you absolutely take time to look into your cosmetics range and skin-care products.

3

Total Hydration Plan

So what can we use water for in the Stay Young Detox? It would almost be easier to ask what we can't use water for. The properties of water are endless. Water is the most common vehicle for cleansing our minds, bodies and spirits. It is also probably the most important, for without water we would die of dehydration within days.

USING WATER IN DETOXIFICATION

Water is a crucial part of detoxification. Detoxification is about cleansing and water is the medium we most commonly use to clean. It is pure, natural and, for most of us, readily available. In many cases of disease or illness, or even when you are just feeling out of sorts, a glass of water is all you may need.

Introducing water into your life on a conscious level will promote your health almost immediately.

9 New Ways to Introduce Water During the 18-day Programme

During the 18-day Stay Young Detox programme you are asked to find 9 new ways to introduce water into your life. Here are some suggestions, but if there is something else that is not here but includes water you can count it in as one of your 9 ways.

Hydration	Drink at least 1.5 litres (3 pints) of water every day.
Urination	Make sure you drink enough for your urine to be clear and odourless.
Colonic irrigation	Introduce a new way of internal cleansing for detoxing inside and out.
Swimming	Get in the swim. Introduce a weekly swim into your life and feel your body totally supported by the water around you.
Thermotherapy	Use the alternating temperature of flowing water to cleanse, tone and invigorate. One simple shower can bring a youthful zest in just moments.
Salt bathing	Use cleansing salts and Epsom salts. Purge your body of toxins and see how it is worth its weight in salt.
Sauna/steam/ Turkish bathing	Use water to wash, sweat out the toxins from within and cleanse the skin at the same time.
Get with the elements	Go to the seaside, breathe in the air and expand your horizons.
Flotation	Use sensory deprivation to make yourself more aware.

Watsu	Go back to the womb, by dancing in water to centre and balance yourself.
Swimming with dolphins	Experience the creatures of the deep and connect to nature through the power of water. Get back to youthful innocence.

Hydration

The first thing you should do every morning and the last thing you should do at night is to drink a glass of water. Just as you wash upon rising and wash before going to bed, drinking water should be thought of from this point on as cleaning your insides. Washing with water is cleaning your outsides. Both are equally important – or you could even say that cleansing within is more important. If you didn't wash you would probably smell after a short period and health risks would only come into play some days later. Not drinking water, however, would result in dehydration and death within just a few days.

Drinking every morning and every evening should be balanced out by drinking continually throughout the day. I don't mean that you should always have a glass to your mouth, but you should average a glass of water an hour, which will eventually add up to 1.5 litres (3 pints) per day – the minimum recommended amount for full hydration. By the end of this section you will probably decide to drink around 2 litres (4 pints) a day over the course of the day.

If you feel thirsty then your body is telling you that you are already beginning to feel dehydrated – so drink some water. Don't ignore the request. Our bodies are incredibly intelligent and only generally ask if they truly do need something.

Look at yourself. If your skin appears dull and lifeless, assess your diet. It is likely that it is less than healthy and that the only fluids going in are coffee, tea or soft drinks. Change these to water, fruit juices (in moderation) and more water. Very soon you will be looking at healthy skin cells, fully hydrated and glowing with vitality.

Don't drink with meals, but drink before you eat – at least half an hour before. Not only will this take the edge off your appetite, but it will also help your body to absorb the nutrients without having to fight through a muddy pile of foodstuffs to find them.

Our bodies are around 75 per cent water, with men having slightly more and women slightly less. We need to keep that level stable. We lose water throughout the day through our skin, our breath and our kidneys. We lose water as we get older – our bodies don't need as much as our metabolism slows down and we don't need as much energy.

We use water in our bodies for cell metabolism. Our cells need to be bathed in water and contain water. The balance must be right or we become out of balance. Our brains are 85 per cent water and the messages in the brain are sent by electrical current – we know that water is a good conductor of electricity, so hydrate your brain and become instantly more intelligent and think at twice the speed!

Water regulates the temperature of our bodies – we sweat if we need to stay cool. This means that we need to drink more water during the warmer months or after exercise or other periods of exertion.

Water keeps the skin moisturised from within. Skin cells can only stay healthy, plump and fresh if there is a good supply of water, since water forms the bulk of the living cell. Our skin therefore needs water for the cells to regenerate. Drinking alcohol and caffeine regularly leads to dehydration of both the body and the skin. Drinking water will balance or rectify this imbalance. Dehydrated skin looks dull, lined, tired, pale and pasty. It is the difference between fresh, plush, smooth and velvety grape versus dried, old, knobbly prune. I know which one I would prefer to have and I am sure that fully hydrated skin keeps us looking younger for a lot longer.

Urination

Water helps aid digestion. It helps food move through the gut, flushes out toxic materials and cleanses the bowel. It prevents kidney stones and helps the body to avoid urinary infections such as cystitis.

Having the correct water balance in the body helps in the achievement of the correct Ph (positive hydrogen) balance. If the Ph is out of balance then our bodies become too acidic or too alkaline, neither of which is safe or desirable. Water replenishes, cleanses, rejuvenates and restores and is probably the most important single item in the detox programme. Do you need any more reasons to take the next sip?

If we drink enough water our urine should consist mainly of concentrated water, clear and odourless. If our urine is dark and strongly perfumed this is a good indication that we need more water. Aim for clear and see how much water it really does take to be fully flushed.

Colonic irrigation

Colonic irrigation has been around since as early as 1500 BC, but seems to be a relatively new and experimental therapy for most people today.

Colonic irrigation consists of an internal bath that helps to cleanse the colon of accumulated poisons, gases, faecal matter and mucous deposits. The practitioner gently pumps filtered water into the rectum and this softens and flushes away any unwanted build-up of toxins and waste.

Colonic irrigation is extremely effective during any detox programme. During the programme you eliminate any source of toxins from your diet. This means that all toxins are being processed and eliminated and not being replaced. There will still be a build-up of toxins within the body from before the programme, which superfoods such as brown rice, nuts and pulses will help to break down. Colonic irrigation will speed up this breakdown and will actively flush out any unwanted/undesirable matter.

The colonic irrigation practitioner asks the person who is being treated to lie on a couch or plinth, with the lower body covered with a towel or sheet. Filtered water at a carefully regulated temperature is introduced under gentle gravitational pressure through the rectum and into the colon. The practitioner uses massage to help the water soften and cleanse the colon of faecal matter and waste, which is flushed away with the waste water. The colon is worked on in stages: each time water is pumped in and flushed out until the whole process is complete. The treatment lasts less than an hour and the modesty of the client is observed throughout – practitioners are totally aware of the 'unusual' circumstances that they place their clients in. It is usual for the practitioner to recommend how many further treatments are required, and also to suggest supplements that will replace natural bowel fibre and flora. The after-effects of colonic irrigation are similar to those of the entire detox programme: a feeling of well-being, lightness, mental clarity, increased energy, loss of bloating, relief from constipation and clearer, glowing skin.

Colonics is not something that normally springs to mind as a complementary therapy – we normally think of massage or aromatherapy – but if you have ever thought about trying this treatment to see what the effects would be, or if you believe that it would help but have never got around to booking a session, then this is the time to try. It's painless, it's different, it makes you feel great and it is detoxifying.

Swimming

If your joints ache or your back is breaking; if you could benefit from some exercise but don't want to run the risk of injury; or if you simply want to feel weightless and graceful, then take yourself off for a swim.

The feeling of water supporting you and taking the pressure off your joints is liberating. Swimming is one of the best ways to exercise without damaging your joints or muscles. You are only working against your own body weight and the resistance of the water. There are no sudden moves and no major impacts. Even just treading water will provide you with good exercise with no element of danger in the form of injury.

Thermotherapy/hydrotherapy

The taking of the waters has long been a tradition in many cultures. Drinking and bathing in water is nothing new. The mineral content of natural waters is highly beneficial. Sebastian Kneipp developed an entire treatment based on the use of hot and cold water. Kneipp was a Dominican priest working in the 18th century in Germany. He developed a theory that water was essential to the body's ability to heal itself. The Kneipp school and spa in Bad Worishhofen in Germany still practise and teach his findings to this day.

We can go to a modern spa and be jetted with water to eliminate cellulite and tone muscles. We can do exercise in a pool and go and get our bodies pummelled and processed in a Turkish bath. Treatments involving water are incredibly beneficial. Treatments involving alternate hot and cold water (*see pages 204–207*) are phenomenally effective.

Salt bathing

There are many treatments that incorporate salts. You can be rubbed by them, wrapped in them and you can even travel to the Dead Sea and swim or float in them. The Dead Sea has such a high concentration of salt that it is impossible to actually go under the surface without making a huge effort. The density of the water makes everything float quite naturally. The salts purge toxins and cleanse the skin. It's a long way to travel but a wonderful experience.

There are ways to use salt bathing at home and Epsom

salts baths (*see also page 213*) are just as effective as many spa treatments.

Magnesium is an essential requirement for nearly all of our cellular activity. Magnesium can be found in high concentration in Epsom salts, which are pure magnesium, and bathing in Epsom salts allows the skin to absorb the magnesium. In addition, the magnesium will absorb or 'draw' toxins from the body, so it is likely that you will 'glow' with perspiration for a while after your bath. This will not be quite a sweat – unless you wrap up really warm!

You are more likely to feel as though you are in a very humid room. It is important to keep warm, not only to increase the effect of the magnesium but also to prevent yourself from catching a chill. Epsom salts baths will improve circulation and speed up the elimination of toxins.

An Epsom salts bath can also be extremely relaxing and warming, helping to soothe aching joints and muscles. Taken before bed this will almost certainly guarantee the deepest night's sleep!

A recipe and instructions are at the back of the book (*see page 213*). Relax and invigorate yourself.

Sauna and steam

The availability of saunas and steam rooms is common. Hotels and gyms are almost guaranteed to have at least one to enjoy, if not both. Saunas use dry heat and steam rooms use wet heat to cleanse and sweat the toxins from the body. The use of heat and thermotherapy is greatly beneficial and very relaxing indeed. If you can combine the two with either a cold shower or a plunge in the pool your treatment will be even more therapeutic – although also a little more enlivening, to say the least. The combination of hot and cold is very healing both internally and emotionally.

The sea

My partner has announced that at some stage in our lives he wants us to live near the sea – overlooking it is, I suspect, the idea. The call of the sea is very common. As far as I know he has never lived near the sea and nor have his parents; he has never worked by the sea and even gets seasick at the merest hint of a rocking boat; but live near the sea he wants to, and he is not alone in this desire. Many hundreds of people move/retire/buy a holiday home or just visit the sea on a regular basis to share its immense intrigue.

Anyone who works with the sea will tell you about the huge respect you need to have for this female. It is only controlled by the moon for tides, and apart from this it is a law unto itself. It can change from a mill pond to a raging, crashing, waved brute in just minutes, and it can take lives in moments if the right care is not taken.

Anyone who thinks they are in charge of this deep, mysterious being can think again. Maybe this is the secret of its therapeutic effect; maybe the gentle ripple of the waves, or the strong crashing of the waves, is what makes us feel mortal and humble. The sea is a product of mother nature and we can just look on it in wonder. It has its own life force; it gives life to a whole different world that has its own laws of the jungle, and it has the mythology of the people from the sea. It is one of the strongest elements and it keeps us guessing. Maybe we will move sooner than we planned.

Flotation

There are two ways to experience a float, but only one good way. There are many 'tanks' that resemble a Reliant Robin in a small room full of water: not as warm as it should be and smelling a tad mustier than we would like. This is not the type to choose. Then there is the version that is exactly the right temperature, is clean and fresh, and has plenty of space available, so that you never come into contact with a fibreglass wall during your float. That is the one to try.

Floating is about sensory deprivation. You cannot feel any part of you and if you get it right you can eventually clear your head of thoughts and just 'be'. The temperature of the water is the same as that of your body, so you cannot feel the water supporting you; there is no light so there is no vision, and there is no sound so there is nothing to hear. Everything has gone and you are left suspended in space, floating on nothing but very safe and comfortable. You are truly divested of everything and taken back to base sensation. It is often likened to being in the womb. What a fabulous way to renew, to invigorate and to emerge to start again.

Watsu

The use of water to support the body while a practitioner takes you through a balletic sequence of moves and stretches is just magical. It combines the flotation experience with gentle exercise and stretches similar to shiatsu massage, and is very sensuous. You are aware of the noises around you and the movement of the water near your ears. You are aware of the body being moved into different positions, gently gliding from one move to another. The stretch is held and then released, and the whole experience feels like a combination of flying and floating. It's truly wonderful and less passive than flotation.

Swimming with dolphins

Many people talk of the wonder of swimming with dolphins or going on a voyage to see the whales swimming in their natural habitat.

There is something mystical about these animals. Dolphins are intelligent and whales are absolutely huge mammals that live in the water. You hear of people who have seen these beautiful creatures and who have said that it has quite fundamentally changed their lives. What a fabulous aid to staying young. It could make you reassess your own life and to put things into perspective, to recapture your own youth.

The actual experience is quite amazing. I have seen dolphins or porpoises swimming alongside a boat only once, when I was on holiday with a big group of friends in Turkey. It was 6.00 a.m. and the crew was shouting and whooping about them. I got up and stumbled onto deck to be totally mesmerised by the sheer beauty, speed and grace of them. You couldn't actually see how they were moving along so fast in front of the bow of the boat. Nothing was wobbling and nothing flapping, and no fins were moving that you could see. Their sheer power and grace were able to propel them with what seemed like no effort whatsoever.

All I do know was that in the time I was watching them, nothing else featured. I was in a place that was the dolphins and me. I had no worries about anything, and was just watching the amazing qualities of nature and appreciating its beauty. It was fabulous fun. It made me want to giggle like a child and it was very exciting – which for me at 6.00 a.m. is pretty incredible in itself, I can assure you.

If you get the chance to make a booking to see dolphins or whales during the 18 days of the programme, then do so. If you don't, file away the idea in your memory stores, and if you ever get the chance, grab it with both hands. This is how to truly enjoy and value life – whatever age you are.

4

Stay Young, Stay Fit Detox

You must take 30 minutes exercise every day or 1 hour every other day – no more and no less.

We all know that exercise is good for us. We hear theories and read articles about some types of exercise being more or less damaging or more or less effective for us, but on the whole there is no denying that exercise is good for us.

If you like exercise and need no prompting, then you are let off this chapter. Just get right on with the sessions each day or every other day. If, like me, you still need forcing into your Lycra read on.

Personally, I am acutely aware of how beneficial exercise is but try as I might, I just cannot enjoy it. I enjoy its effects – fitness, vitality, energy, toned arms, fresh-looking skin and much, much more – but it still doesn't mean I like it.

However, like it or not you have no excuse: exercise is one of the best ways to promote the Stay Young Detox programme. Exercise is also one of the means of actually physically reversing the signs of ageing.

WHY EXERCISE IS GOOD FOR YOU

As we get older and less fit, our muscles begin to deteriorate. This happens gradually and quite normally without regular exercise. If we start to introduce exercise into our life, and especially into our 18-day detox programme, then we can grow our muscles younger. Working on the fibres will make them respond as if they are younger: they will be more toned, more elastic, more flexible and more able to heal after injury. Exercise can actually shorten the time between muscle damage and muscle repair, and the fitter body is able to get physically better more quickly than the unfit body.

Exercise increases blood flow, circulation, the heart rate, and the metabolism of the internal organs, and increases and/or balances cell and hormone production. Exercise balances the pH of the body; it tones the muscles and tightens the skin and makes us glow with vitality. It is also free if we choose it to be – there really is no excuse not to introduce regular exercise into your life.

The UK Fitness Association lists dozens of benefits to exercise, but the following are the most relevant to the Stay Young programme. Exercise preserves muscle, improves memory function, circulation and mental agility, prevents osteoporosis, lessens arthritis pain, lowers blood pressure and lowers cholesterol. The list goes on but in short, the conclusion is that exercise actually lengthens life.

The good thing about exercise is that it has an almost immediate effect. Regular exercise encourages the body to produce a feel-good factor hormone – serotonin – which will mean that you may even look forward to more exercise, or at least a regular exercise routine.

The best thing to do is to work out for yourself what sort of exercise you are most likely to enjoy, be able to do according to your body's ability, and be able to do regularly in conjunction with your current lifestyle. Attempting to totally change the way you operate in order to fit in hours at the gym is at best difficult and at worst impossible to achieve, as well as being totally demotivating.

What do you like doing that could also be construed as exercise?

- Walking in the country.
- Walking in the city.
- Walking the dog.
- Playing in the garden with the children.
- Playing a sport with friends or partner.
- Working out in a gym.
- Hiring and working out with a personal trainer.
- Working out with a shared personal trainer.
- Going to Salsa classes.
- Going to Siroc classes.
- Doing heavy-duty gardening.
- Swimming.
- Rock climbing.
- Night clubbing.

The list can be endless and if you can find a method that 'disguises' the fact that you are exercising, you may be more likely to stick to the 18-day plan and beyond – exercise is not just for Christmas.

You don't necessarily have to do the same exercise every time. Look at the list and if several types of exercise look interesting try them all, add some of your own and alternate. Variety is the key to keeping your interest, and if you can do something that you absolutely cannot see yourself doing that may be the exact thing to start with.

There are, of course, the more traditional methods of exercising, going to the gym, for example. Joining a gym can be very expensive and you don't want to become one of the many who make gym owners rich by simply donating a monthly payment to somewhere you have only seen once in your life. (You would get more benefit from donating the funds to your favourite charity.) A simple exercise sequence for toning your whole body, which you can easily carry out at home, is included at the back of this book (*see pages 217–218*).

You should also think about how you start your exercise sensibly. If you have never done anything remotely active, putting on some old trainers and jogging around the block could actually be dangerous for you. Exercise doesn't have to be hot and sweaty before it is beneficial. We know that sweat is the currency for hard exercise, but some types of exercise can work very well in different ways.

If you are beginning with a gym or trainer it is likely that the person assigned to you will take a full body check and advise a plan of action. If you go to a class you will be watched as a beginner, so you will be in no danger of overdoing it. If you choose to exercise by yourself, however, you must be aware of some basic rules.

Start very slowly. Do some exercise for about 5 minutes, then stretch your muscles. Stretching when the muscles are totally cold can be as damaging as not stretching at all. Build up the time you exercise over a period of days. Don't go straight in with one full hour of high-impact running or jogging. The first half hour can be something as simple as walking continuously around your garden or home. Just do enough to bring your pulse rate up to higher than it is normally. Slow down what you are doing in the last 5 or 10 minutes of your chosen time. Stretch at the end of your session.

Whatever your chosen exercise method you should try and make it enjoyable, different and varied. Recognise how beneficial the exercise is for you and how simple it is to feel young and vital.

5

Indulgence Programme

The wonderful thing about being slightly more mature is that you can be immature; in addition, you will have worked out by now exactly what you like.

Indulgences are special and essential. In order to stay perfectly young we must be able to indulge ourselves. It is our reward for getting as far as we have. There is not much that I need to say in this section except that you cannot leave it out. The worst thing you can do to ruin your Stay Young Detox is to dip on the indulgences. I have compiled a list of some obvious choices of things you could indulge in, but you can substitute them with something else if you really want to – that is your indulgence.

There are no details following the indulgences; they speak for themselves. They should happen every day.

The Indulgences

You should choose only one indulgence a day, but you may opt for the same one every day if this is your preference. You should not exceed your quota of indulgences, but you absolutely must enjoy them!

Drinking a 150 ml glass of good red wine	Full of antioxidants; a positive rejuvenator.
Eating chocolate: 4 squares of dark chocolate consisting of at least 70 per cent minimum cocoa solids	Full of antioxidants: again, essential nutrition.
Having a long soak in a bath by candlelight	Bathe your body to beauty and youth. Prevent all interruptions and just sink under the weight of the indulgence. No children, no calls, no nothing except you.
Reading a magazine from cover to cover	Curl up on the sofa, forbid any disturbance and read the junk – how frivolous and shallow. Just brilliant!
Going for coffee	Take yourself away from it all. Take time out to have a properly made, real coffee, a hot one, not one cooled by other people's demands.
Drinking a 150 ml glass of champagne	This needs no explanation; it's the elixir of gods – and goddesses.

Having a facial, manicure or pedicure	Have one, have them all. Let someone else take the years away and make you feel perfectly primped.
Having a lie in	Stay in bed for at least an hour after your normal time. See how much it throws everyone out. Let them appreciate you while you are indulging yourself. Emerge refreshed and relaxed.

As you indulge yourself, read the following and see how it makes so much sense. To stay sane, young and alive we need to make sure we look after ourselves. It shouldn't be an option; it should be an essential requirement.

'IF THE COOKIE JAR IS EMPTY THEN YOU CAN'T GIVE THEM COOKIES.'

Imagine yourself as a cookie jar. The jar is full of a freshly baked selection of different types of cookie: chocolate chip, ginger, orange spice, cinnamon, white chocolate, blueberry, raisin, walnut, coffee and oatmeal. They are warm, highly nutritious – despite their yumminess! – and simply delicious. You also love these cookies because you actually baked them yourself with your own hands. You feel fulfilled because you have created something and now you can share it with anyone who wants it.

Letting people tuck into these cookies is immensely pleasing. Their hands lift the lid. The smell is wonderful and gets the taste buds stimulated. The texture is crunchy and crumbly, and the flavour travels from the mouthwatering first bite right through the body until the last crumb. They are pleasing and satisfying. They fill you up and they provide nutrition to help you carry on for the rest of the day.

As the cookies are eaten and enjoyed, you are able to replace them by simply baking a new batch each evening and then placing this in your own personal jar. This is not tiring because it gives you pleasure to bake and also to see how much everyone that tastes the cookies enjoys them. You and your life are in cookie heaven.

Now, several weeks later your cookies have gained a reputation. They are still everything they were before, and you still put as much love and attention into them, but they are going faster and faster. As fast as they are being eaten you have a job to keep up replacing them. Your oven isn't big enough to bake the batch sizes you need to, and the hands are dipping into the jar without even taking the time to taste the cookies. Some people are even taking a handful of cookies and passing them out to friends! It is OK, though, because the cookies are still of a high standard. Everyone is getting a top-notch cookie and no one would ever know that you are exhausted because it is taking you much more time to replenish the rapidly disappearing stocks. You need some time off because every time they lift the lid and reach for a cookie, you have made sure that there are plenty of cookies to go around – despite the damage to your own health and quality of life.

Six months after the first taste of a cookie the troops are getting restless. The jar is not always full, or when it is it only has one or two flavours available. Some of the cookies are a little overcooked or, worse still, a touch too soggy. You have resorted to getting up early to fit more baking in, and you are going to bed tired because you have to spend more of your time deciding on new flavours or new shapes of cookie to keep them happy. To keep your sanity you make a decision to make one flavour and hope that this will satisfy all. You also decide to make just a few. If they run out, then so be it; if they go stale, then so be it. Now you realise that you don't bake with loving care and attention, you simply bake to satisfy the demand for the cookie – they are not even your cookies anymore, but have become public property.

The cookie eaters can taste all these changes and they don't like them. 'Why can't we have cookies like we used to?' 'Why can't we have all the flavours?' 'Why aren't there enough?' 'Why don't you like baking them anymore?' 'What has gone wrong?' **'Why is the cookie jar empty?'**

If you map the cookie jar theory out on your own life, then it begins to sound all too familiar. If you do not feel fully replenished, satisfied and fully stocked, you do not have the resources to give out help, time and understanding to other people. If you are exhausted, giving your remaining energy away to other people will leave you depleted and drained. If no one is putting back into your cookie jar then how can you offer cookies to anyone else? The best person to put back into your jar is YOU. You can replenish, revive, invigorate, sort, eliminate, satisfy and grow yourself because you are the only person who truly knows what you do and don't want to happen in your life.

The Stay Young Detox will hopefully make you realise how important you are to the way you think and feel. Youth is a state of mind and if you feel and think young,

PART **2**

Your Mind

Introduction

The Stay Young Detox tackles the subject of staying young from all angles, whether they be concerned with the physical or the mental. If we think of ourselves as old, or have this notion that certain things should be done at certain ages, then whatever we eat or do our thoughts will still prevent us from experiencing all the fabulous things that life has to offer – at any age!

Getting our heads straight about what is and isn't important will help us see that with the right attitude we can achieve anything we want to, small or large, significant or insignificant.

This section looks at:

• Getting your life in balance.

• Getting a positive outlook.

• Looking at ways to grow yourself.

You should complete one of the exercises from each of the 3 mind steps detailed in this section every other day of the programme.

Getting your thoughts and life into balance will give

everything a place and a time. If everything is out of balance, you will be constantly juggling, not knowing what should happen, when, why or how. Sound familiar?

Being able to turn everything to a positive means that you can get everything to work in your favour. Nothing need be against you anymore. This may come as a surprise or shock and it may not initially be welcome, but it certainly can be changed to a positive over time, and that will become a benefit.

Growing yourself is something you probably have never considered. Physically we grow all the time – we may even grow more than we might necessarily want to, but we grow nevertheless. When we are young we go to school, and every day is a learning and growing experience. As soon as we reach so-called adulthood, we stop allowing ourselves time to grow. We give our time to others so that they can grow; we help others so that they have time to do things that will grow them, but we often don't seem to make time for our own growth.

The three subjects described in this section are incredibly important to us. The Stay Young Detox is about cleansing our lives of the detrimental aspects and putting in or sticking to the beneficial aspects. We perceive that staying young is an age thing. It is in part, but it is also a huge head thing. If we think old, then we will think we shouldn't do things at our age. We will think that we are too old or that we have missed the chance. However, if we actually change the way we think about ourselves we can pretty much see that we can actually do anything we want to at our age because we have the wisdom, knowledge and experience that we previously didn't have – in fact it would be nigh on careless to have attempted some things at any age except this one! We certainly won't have missed any chances, as we now have the knowledge to make the best out of every situation, so much so that we now make our own chances and grow our own luck. We are never too old unless there is no breath in our bodies.

There are 3 steps in each chapter in this section – 9 in total. Each day you carry out a task that makes you look at yourself, your life or your thoughts differently, or you do something that makes you feel differently. Getting a new perspective on your own life gives you the chance to see if you are getting what you want and what you need out of your life. We use our minds continually, so if there are thoughts like 'too old' or 'not for me' that are jumbled, confused or just not straight, then anything that can sort them through and put them in some form of order will help.

Usually we only take a long, hard look at ourselves when something has gone wrong, or when someone actually tells us to in the heat of an argument. The result is that we generally resolve to be a better person – for at least a day!

The Stay Young Detox programme requires you to actually stop and take a really long look, not just at yourself, but inside yourself and all around yourself. You can be completely private. You may wish to write things down on a day-to-day basis or you may wish to simply use your mind.

The Stay Young Detox requires a clear-thinking mind. Part of looking at yourself is being truthful about what you want in life – not just in the areas of health, wealth and happiness (join the queue!), but also in regard to much more specific things, which can be achieved more immediately. Keeping your eye on the big picture is very important, but you have to have the smaller, more immediate pictures coloured in to keep you going. You will be asked to *think* about what you really desire – desire is better than want because it injects a real passion and passion is a strong motivational tool. It doesn't ask what you desire at your age; it asks what you truly desire. Do you desire to try things you think have been beyond you before? Do you desire to replan the garden? Do you desire to have more or fewer friends? Do you desire to go out more? If you sort the 'small picture' desires, then the big picture comes along quite naturally. Several of the tasks suggested below will help you sort through the pile of day-to-day frivolous ideas and find the true desires and let you focus and develop them.

LIVING FOR THE MOMENT

Planning for the future is very, very important, but don't wish your life away! Living for the moment is great fun. You get loads more out of each day without doing anything other than living your life and feeling how it feels instead of just doing what you have to do. Living for the moment means thinking for the moment, so think about things you can do today, today, and leave thinking about things you cannot do until tomorrow, until tomorrow.

If you don't organise your brain to work this way, then before you know it you will be thinking about everything that gets in the way of doing what you want to do and a million reasons why you shouldn't do it – and really, the only thoughts we should ever have are 'how?' not 'if'. If we always thought this way we would never actually get on with 'doing' anything. You should also learn to let your mind relax and regenerate, actually plan to do nothing and do things for no reason. Don't, however, just let time slip away unnoticed – use it as relaxation, so that when you want to think about something you are ready to. Then, when you want to do something, you can just make the arrangements, not think about why you shouldn't be doing it.

THE BIG CLEAR-OUT

Our minds are fantastic at retaining all the information we have learnt, we need, we create, and that's very important for day-to-day life. We are also good at holding on to things we don't need, both physically and, more importantly, mentally. We bear grudges, get niggled that someone has something we don't, get annoyed that the bus didn't arrive on time yesterday, worry that the bus won't even come on Thursday, and so on and so on. The Stay Young Detox will look at ways to sort out the things you can do something about – and make you do them – and also the things that you cannot do anything about and make you forget, sort or file them safely to a more suitable time, or not let them get in the way. Worrying about doing something that you think you shouldn't do, worrying about something that may never happen or has happened, is exhausting and wastes energy. *Doing* something to stop you worrying and start you enjoying whatever you want to enjoy is exhilarating and a brilliant use of your time.

WHO AM I?

Are you true to your self? The only way to be true to your self is to know who is the real you. What does your mind think about your body? What do *you* think about your mind? What do *you* think about your body? Are they all the same? Do you separate them, and do you 'feel' or do you 'do'? Are you what other people think you are? Have you bowed down to this age thing? Is there another side that hasn't been let out for fear of shocking other people, or do you deliberately go out of your way to cause a stir? Can you change bits of you that you don't want, and can you enhance bits you really like?

Each and every task in the programme will help you on your way to understanding and discovering something about yourself. Once the tasks have been completed you will know yourself. You will know how you feel and what you want in life, and how to start to go about getting it. You will know how to just do stuff, to live in the moment; know how to clear out your personal junk and to keep hold of the bits you like and use them to your advantage.

It won't be easy. There will be days that are exhausting due to the fact that you will be using your mind in a way that it hasn't been used for years – a breath of fresh air always makes you more tired but it is a healthy tired, a tired that was truly earned, not born out of boredom and tedium. Clearing your mind will stop you worrying unnecessarily and stop you stressing over things that are just thoughts and never actually reality. A 'stay young' mind will be clear of everything but the essential or enjoyable.

6

Stay In Balance Detox

TALK TO YOURSELF

On the day you choose to do this exercise you must take time out to get to know your 'self'. You may think that this is odd. Given that you are your 'self', surely you know everything about you that there is to know. This is true but as with so many things, it is taken for granted: you take your 'self' for granted.

Every day you carry out tasks, jobs and roles, and this is done without question – but how do you really feel about them? Have you listened to your body and found out how it feels? Do you know how you really feel about your diet, your figure, your mind, your exercise regime, your daily routine, etc., etc.?

What I mean about talking to yourself is really listening to yourself and then finding a response – starting a dialogue. If we took time to listen to our own response a lot of things that we do would not be done or would be done differently. If someone calls and says that they need your help to look after their children for a day – you immediately say 'Yes, no problem'. If you stopped to think and listen to yourself you may have found that actually you have a very busy day and it would suit you more if you jointly decided on a solution/date/entertainment for everyone's kids that suited everybody.

If you think you need to go to the gym to keep fit, you pack a bag and toddle off to your next workout. On some occasions, if you actually listened to your body, you could find that it would rather have waited until tomorrow. Your muscles will have had the time to recover from yesterday's workout and your mind would feel much more energetic. Exercise *now* would be a trial – something you had to get through, but exercise *tomorrow* would be invigorating and a great tonic.

Note that listening to yourself should not be an excuse to never do the things you hate, but need doing!!! If you really listened you would know they had to be done.

Listening to yourself should also give you a much more in-depth understanding of how you feel about yourself. For the Stay Young Detox programme you need to start to listen to yourself in a slightly different way, a way that will get you into the habit of listening thoroughly in the future. Writing to yourself really works and the letters will completely surprise you.

Write a letter to yourself about how you feel – be your own penfriend. Your letter could be something along the lines of:

I am really looking forward to the weekend but it seems as if I just get to Friday, collapse because I am tired and before I know it, it is Sunday evening again without my even noticing the weekend.

It would be nice to cancel everything and just rest. I

know the pressure is to get things done, but sooner or later getting things done will turn into pure survival, I am tired and need to make time for me.

Once you have written to yourself, you should always give your body the chance to respond. This was the response that the hypothetical individual above might have felt their body would write as a result of receiving the letter:

This is good. I do need a rest, but I don't need to stop everything. What I would really enjoy is a session in a beauty salon, with a pedicure, manicure and exfoliation, topped off with a glass of wine and a take-away. I will then be refreshed and feel as if I actually spent time on me.

The result could be that the relentless tussle this individual was having between enjoying herself and not becoming exhausted would be resolved simply by taking the time to find out what would actually replenish her stocks. As a consequence, there would be loads of space in her life to get on with other things – she had cleared the fug out of her head.

EXERCISE   Preparation for talking to yourself

You will need a quiet, warm room for an hour, and a pad and pen. You may like to have a tape of relaxation music; make sure it is only music as lyrics are likely to interfere with your thoughts.

In order to get the best out of 'talking to yourself' you

should precede your session with a relaxation exercise. The whole process should take you no more than an hour, but it is important to include the relaxation as you will get much much more out of it.

For the programme you will be writing a broad-ranging letter, a letter that tells your 'self' how you are feeling, what you want to feel, what's causing concerns and what is good – basically anything that is currently in your head and going around in your mind, and what is stopping you feeling as vital as you have been in the past.

Now, lie in a comfortable position, with your back flat on the floor/bed/mat or, if you have back problems, place a cushion under your thighs and knees and this will naturally support your back. Place your arms loosely by your sides and let your legs flop open; make sure that your shoulders are relaxed and your neck is straight. To ensure that everything is relaxed, start by scrunching every muscle in your body as tightly as possible. Hold it for the count of 4, then let everything relax into the floor. Now you need to check that you are breathing correctly to get the best out of the exercise.

To breathe correctly, you simply relax your stomach muscles, inhale slowly through your nose, and take in the air until it feels as if the base of your stomach is full of air. Pause momentarily and then exhale through the mouth. By feeling the air 'in your stomach', you will have relaxed your diaphragm muscle, which means that your lungs have fully expanded and you have inhaled to full capacity. This will feel strange at first but will soon become the normal way to breathe and you won't need to think about it any more.

Now is the time to start to write. Take a pen and write

a letter to your self. Be very honest – if you feel bad put all that in, and if you feel good, put all that in, too. If you like something, then say so and if you hate something, then say so. Don't try and interpret how you are feeling. Just tell it like it is, now, today. Remember – no one will ever see this letter. It is yours alone.

Once you have completed the letter, sit back and do some breathing, then read it back to yourself slowly. The letter will deserve a response. Write back and write how you feel after reading the letter. It was written to you, so how do you feel about it? Does it surprise you or shock you? Have you found out about feelings you didn't know you had, or uncovered irrelevant niggles, or have you discovered important things to work with? Do you know what's making you feel more jaded?

Once you have completed this exercise you will be different. You will have found out more about how you are, and will have cleared out the things you now think are irrelevant and kept the things you have decided are important. You won't have solved all your situations, but you will be able to view them from a new perspective. You will know what you have to work on.

SOME TIME FOR YOURSELF

It is very easy to spend money on entertainment or on keeping yourself occupied without even thinking. It is very easy to think we deserve something special, so we go and spend lots of money on something. When we were young we didn't have much money. We made our own fun, and didn't pay to go anywhere. We spent time with friends on bikes or in gardens.

Now we wake up and think: 'What should I/we do today?' One of the major considerations is the amount of money we have. If we have a lot – it is the start of the month – then we have more choice than at the end of the month, when funds are running low. If we have no money because we are out of work we tend to think we cannot do anything, and if we have had a windfall or a win on the lottery(!), then we can do absolutely anything. Having money to do things and to pay for things stops us from thinking about every option we do have. We tend to ignore the simple and straightforward options and go for the more complicated ones. We have learnt that we can only have fun if we have money. This is not true. If we put in a bit more thought and use our heads, there are millions of things that can be done to keep ourselves occupied, to learn new things or entertain ourselves, which cost nothing. Be more like children, play more like children, be innovative.

For one whole day on the programme you are forbidden the short cuts to happiness and you must actually put in some thought as to how to spend your time without spending any money.

Use the local papers that are delivered to your house, and the local bus and train timetables. This is where they come into their own. Check out sources such as the local post office window, council offices, social centre and the sports centre noticeboard. You will need to collect together all these sources of information. The only other things available to you will be £5.00 per adult, £3.00 per child and your imagination. The money available is really only for emergencies – you win extra points if you do not spend anything during the day.

Planning and spontaneity are key. You will need to really use your mind to find substitutes for the normal 'costly' activities we engage in to pass our spare time or time off. You should do things on the spur of the moment.

To give you an idea of what you can and cannot do, here is a simple list of things you may not do as they will or are costing you money, or involve not using any form of imagination or brain power. 'Use it or lose it' is very relevant when entertaining yourself. If you never think about how you use your time, it will just slip away and you will be old before your time and won't have anything to show for it.

Usual activities no longer permitted:

- Watching television.
- Going to the cinema.
- Dining out.
- Shopping.
- Going on a holiday.
- Driving anywhere.
- Meeting friends for coffee.
- Buying ice creams.
- Going to the leisure centre.
- Having a pub lunch.

Activities that cost nothing and are very definitely permitted include:

- Having a long bath, relaxing and doing lots of home beauty treatments, for example placing tea bags or cucumber slices on your eyes, and having salt scrubs and cold showers.

- Making a cake/having friends round for dinner/lunch using foods from the cupboard.

- Weeding the garden.

- Going for a walk or hike around your town/area.

- Tidying out a room/tidying out a cupboard.

- Looking around a local church/museum/gallery that has free entrance.

- Checking the local papers for outdoor craft fairs to visit – but not buying anything!

- Attending talks at the local town hall that don't require an entrance fee.

- Finding out where your local library is and going and reading about anything you wish to.

- Doing two days of voluntary work.

- Sorting out all your old clothes and delivering them to a local charity shop.

- Putting all your photographs in an album, or at least sorting them out and throwing away all the shots that are out of focus or too dark to see what is actually in the shot.

- Reading a book.

- Visiting a friend whom you haven't seen in ages but who lives within walking distance.

- Sewing buttons on to everything that has lost a button which you've never got around to sewing back on.

And so on and so on – the list of things that cost nothing is much longer and much more interesting than the list of things that would cost you money.

Important things to remember:

- Try to do only minimal preparation – collect the papers and timetables but don't look at them until the morning of your chosen day. This will mean that you will have to use your mind more to come up with something interesting or productive to do.

- If you think about the day too much in advance you may inadvertently get things into the house that will help you entertain yourself – the challenge to your self is to come up with things on the spur of the moment – a genuine case of 'What shall I do today?'.

- Try and remain as sociable as normal. Don't think that you have to become a recluse just because you have no funds – encourage your friends to participate in your challenge. They should be your entertainment, not just people that you spend money with.

- Make a mental note of how you react to having no funds available. Is it unnerving or a challenge? Do you talk more to friends than you normally would or is it the same? Do you look at things differently? Is it more tiring having to use your mind to entertain yourself, or is it more uplifting? Have you got things done that have been hanging around for ever, or did you use your time to try out totally new things?

Ask yourself if you will try this again in the future, or if you think the way you spend your spare time is fulfilling enough. Are you using money instead of your imagination? Are you spending your life away?

TAKE YOURSELF ON RETREAT

Today should be a day off work, a weekend or a holiday, for you will spend it in total silence.

Getting to know what is in your head, what you are thinking and how you are reacting, is very easy if you are not interacting with anyone. If the only dialogue you have all day is with yourself you can find out a lot about yourself. It is like being locked in a room with one person of whom you are free to ask any question you wish – very telling and quite intense, but you will get answers to many of the questions asked.

There are many places that call themselves 'retreats', places where people – who are often religious – can go to stay for a time of reflection or prayer. You do not enter into conversation with anyone on retreat, so whatever your reasons for being there will remain with you. You can re-create these retreat surroundings in your own home and spend your time thinking for yourself, writing lists, writing letters and sorting things out physically, emotionally or mentally.

You will need to prepare for this day by shutting yourself off from the outside world and any outside stimulus. Put the answerphone on or unplug the telephone. Lock the front door and do not answer it. Do not open the post, switch on the radio, television or video recorder, or read newspapers or books. Make sure the day is a full 24 hours from, say, 11.00 p.m. the night before until 11.00 p.m. on the day of your retreat. Many of these hours will be while you are asleep and, indeed, if you use your retreat day to catch up on lost sleep that will be very useful.

Get dressed in something loose, warm and comfortable. If you need to catch up on sleep, then sleep in until you wake, get up and dress. If you need more sleep you can go back to bed for rest as and when required during the day. For the rest of your retreat time you should do things that are not normal. Don't try to do all the household chores and catch up with tidying the house. Retreat should be about you. It should allow you to touch base with yourself, maybe even for the first time ever. You can visit yourself at home.

You may discover that this is the first time you can recall that you spent on your own. Even though you will spend a lot of time on your own, keeping to the rule of silence may make you think about yourself more. Use the day to answer any questions you have for yourself. If you have any problems with relationships, use the time to think through all your options. If you need to decide about your job – not about a problem at work, but about yourself in the context of work – think this through. The fact that you cannot communicate with the outside world means that if you reach a decision you will have the discipline to live with the decision for several hours before you tell anyone. This may give you more time to reflect and to confirm if the decision is right or wrong for you. If there is a lot going on in your life, your day of silence may simply serve to 'let the contents settle' before you carry on with business as usual. We file thoughts in our head so that we can access them at a later date; this filing process can take place when you are relaxing. Kids spend hours just pondering and dreaming. Ponder your most important issues like a child and process them like an adult.

If you believe that you are very straight and organised in your head, and that there is nothing you would like time to think about or think through, then well done. (What's your secret!?) Seriously, even if you have everything sorted you should still 'retreat' and use the time for deep relaxation exercises, correct breathing and doing nothing. Doing nothing is extremely hard. Listen to your breathing, feel your heartbeat through your body and become aware of every aspect of your mind and body.

Important things to remember:

You must not do anything that involves stimulus from outside, for retreat is about you and your own mind. A good view out of the window of country, sky or garden (but no streets or people) is all you are permitted. If the views from your retreat include traffic or people, look inwards at your own house and cut off the outside world. If something distracts you, just let it pass. Don't dwell on it and return to your own thoughts.

Awake feeling refreshed and invigorated and armed with the clear thinking of a revived mind.

7

Thinking Yourself Young Detox

SMILING WHEN THE GOING GETS TOUGH

It seems a shame that something so simple as smiling – which even children can manage to do without thinking 400 times a day – sometimes seems to be so hard for adults. We get out of the habit of smiling as there is so much else to think about, so much else that is serious and doesn't warrant a smile. If you look at it another way, it would be so much better to do a lot of the serious stuff with a smile. If you are asking someone to do something, smiling makes the task seem so much easier or positive. If you smile when doing a task, the task seems lighter and less arduous; if you frown the task becomes yet another thing on the long list of things you have to get done.

Meeting someone with a 'friendly' or 'happy' smile makes us want to smile back, and it makes us feel good, too. If we have a laugh or something makes us giggle, then everything seems to become less severe, less problematic.

So today, you should think about your smile.

- Smile at your neighbour and say good morning or hello with a big smile.

- Greet the first person you meet in the street with a smile.

- When you pick up the phone, say your number or name with a smile.

- If someone opens a door for you, say thank you and smile.

- If you need to read anything or go through a document, make sure you exchange a dour, serious look for a smile – it will make the reading that much more interesting.

- Write your diary with a smile; think of all the fabulous things you have done and the people you have met. Smile and a normal, everyday task will become a joy.

Smiling is contagious; there is nothing more likely to make you giggle than someone who is giggling uncontrollably themselves. There is nothing more likely to make you smile than someone giving you a great big grin. Find something on a daily basis that will let you have a little chuckle to yourself.

The main thing to remember when it comes to smiling is that you have to mean it. If you sit in front of a mirror first thing in the morning or during the evening of the day before your 'smile-in' and simply make the shape of a smile you will see that it looks awful. You will also recognise it as the sort of smile you get from tired shop assistants or from someone who truly doesn't want to smile, but feels that they have to at least look a bit happier. No, a smile needs to be sincere. A real smile will light up your face, crinkle your eyes and wrinkle your nose; it will show your teeth and lift your cheeks; and it will make you feel great. So try it out a few times, mainly to remind yourself just how good you look when wearing a smile; then you will be fully prepared for the day ahead.

Remember that the smile must be genuine.

At the end of the day, write down a few words about how you felt about smiling all day. Was it exhausting or uplifting? Did it feel strange at first or did it feel natural? Did you enjoy it? Did it make you smile?

FIND ROOM TO THINK GOOD

We all have ghosts or skeletons in our minds. We are full of 'What if?', 'I wonder if?', 'I should have' and 'If only'. We get wrapped up in the seriousness of our own lives.

If we use our time more effectively, do something about our worries instead of just worrying, we can clear a lot more space and create a lot more peace in our minds. They say that children have good imaginations, but when it comes to worrying about what may never happen, adults win hands down.

Because we believe there is nothing we can do to sort out a situation, we keep going over and over it in our minds, using valuable space that would be better taken up with doing something positive and constructive rather than with negative and destructive things.

Today we can clean those negative thoughts away or file them so that they can be used when we choose to use them rather than having them spring to mind when we least need them to.

EXERCISE Clearing your mind

The first step is to note down all the things that you truly believe you cannot do anything about but want to resolve in order to clear them from your thoughts. Also note down the things that really take up space in your head, which you want to do something about but have not acted upon.

Now you can start to make amends and clear your mind:

- Taking the situations and/or individuals one at a time, write them a letter.

- Make sure that you cover every issue that concerns you and that you put in the letter exactly how you feel about the situation; put down all your emotions.

- Include anything that has resulted from a situation or incident that is on your mind, and any repercussions that have occurred since then.

- Take every thought from your mind and write it down.

Whatever you decide to do with the letters, store them, burn them, read them or even send them, you can rest assured that all your unsettled business will now be settled. All your thoughts will have been faced and sorted – they won't have gone away, but they will now have been managed and you should feel really positive that you have taken some action.

In future make sure that you 'sort' your thoughts before they get too disruptive. If you can say what you feel, then say it right on the spot so that it doesn't fester. If you don't want to say it, write a letter immediately, saying how you feel and send it – the sooner you write the less you will have to say because you won't have had time to dwell on the issue and make a mountain out of a mole hill. Make sure, however, that you do think before you write, as once the letter has been sent – it has been said!

Writing your thoughts down in a letter addressed to them will enable you to say anything to anyone, any time. The sooner you get your thoughts down on paper the sooner they will stop spinning around in your head.

PERCEIVED RISK TAKING

If anything concentrates the mind it is a small dose of abject terror! Moreover, as you go through the 'my whole life flashed before me' bit you also get to take a long look at yourself. That is incredibly interesting – you find out so much about yourself and how you feel, and how you react, in just a few short moments.

The Stay Young Detox is not about putting you at risk – far from it. It is about looking at things differently so that you can clear your mind of the rubbish and keep the important stuff. Putting yourself through an extreme experience (with all safety measures observed so there is no actual risk – only a perceived one) is a very concise way to find out what is important to you.

Perceived risks can be taken by going along to a place where there are professionals ready and equipped to take you through an experience while observing all the correct safety rules and guidelines and also assessing if you are fit and able to carry out the task without putting yourself in any danger. The risk will be all in your head, and your ability to carry out the task will be your own personal ability to 'get your head around' something you wouldn't normally dream of doing.

The sorts of things we are talking about are:

- Parachute jump

- Rock climbing

- Flying an aircraft

- White-water rafting

- Balloon flight

- Glider flight

- Holding an insect or reptile

- Mountain biking

- Exploring caves

- Bidding at an auction

- Scuba diving

- Public speaking

It is hard to name everything that would fit into this

category but you need to find something that would truly be a massive thing for you to do. (In fact, anything that you consider you are too old to do could be on this list.)

Important things to remember:

- Do something that will really challenge you and test your comfort zone.

- Don't listen to anyone else's opinion about what they think would be the most terrifying thing. Work it out for yourself and then, when you feel ready to start, make the necessary arrangements.

- Call the association or club that operates the 'risk of your choice' and find out as much as you feel you need to know.

- Once you have found something that you would like to have a go at and that fits your budget and your timing, just go ahead and book it.

Obviously, this is a lot to get done in one day, but you should be able to start to think through the project – and work out the best time to schedule your risk taking. Good luck and fingers crossed!

8

Growing Young Detox

TEACH YOURSELF SOMETHING NEW

Choose an appliance that you have never really understood, something that you have refused to master under
the heading of 'I'm too old for that new-fangled stuff' – or
perhaps 'I'm technophobic'. Banish such excuses forever.
You could, for instance, try:

- Using the video recorder.

- Using the deep fat fryer, juicer or food processor – but
  watch those fingers.

- Setting the memory on the telephone.

- Trying the delicates wash on the washing machine.

- Storing names on your mobile phone.

- Setting up the answerphone service on your mobile
  phone.

- Checking the oil and water in the engine of your car.

- Setting the timer on the central heating thermostat.

- Learning to wire a plug.

- Programming the padlock on a suitcase.

Once you have chosen the appliance, select a function that to date has been pushed to the back of your mind, or alternatively has always been labelled as someone else's job – or placed in the category of 'Life's too short to know how to tune the VCR' – and quite simply, teach yourself how to do it. A manual should take you through a step-by-step sequence to reach your goal. If at first you don't succeed, breathe deeply and try again.

Important things to remember:

Make sure you have all the relevant parts that the manual describes. If a vital piece is missing or broken, then no matter how you try, you will probably find it impossible to get any results and this will be very unsatisfying indeed.

Make sure you find something that you want to solve. If you never use the video or never need to set the timer on the oven, you will gain little satisfaction from learning the process – choose, instead, say to programme your telephone with all your most often used numbers.

Make a mental note of how your task will make your life easier and less complicated. You could, for instance:

- Watch more good television as you can now record important programmes that clash with others.

- Have more time to yourself on Sundays and still enjoy a full Sunday roast.

- Call all your friends and tell them your news.

- Replenish the water for your windscreen without having to pull into a service station during a long journey or, more importantly, never run out of oil and ruin your engine.

- Reduce your car 'rescue' premium by never having to call out a driving organisation.

- Come home to a wonderfully warm house in the middle of winter.

- Open your suitcase knowing that it still holds its original contents.

You should also make a mental note of other things that you could do in the technical field to make your life easier – and make a date to do them.

CREATIVE THINKING

Do something different; feel uncertain about something but go for it nonetheless; swap things around and see how it feels. Get a fresh, new perspective.

- I always get up at the same time.

- I always have the same thing for breakfast.

- I go into my office.

- I have lunch at the same time every day.

- I finish work at the same time every day.

- I go home from the office every day.

- I watch television.

- I make the supper.

- I get up at the same time every day.

Does this sound familiar? If it does, it means that you are set in your ways.

There is no room in such a lifestyle for any creativity. I know what happens and when it happens during my day. I have no need to think about anything because it just happens that way. Now, if I were to change everything I do around – I would need to keep my wits about me about when and if everything would get done.

Your day of change should be total. Everything you do should be done differently. Choose a day that would have been completely run of the mill and turn it upside down:

- Set the alarm earlier or later.

- Get out of the other side of the bed.

- Have your shower/bath before breakfast or after breakfast, whichever is not the norm.

- Get dressed in a completely different outfit.

- If you usually wear dark colours choose anything you have that is bright and vice versa.

- If you normally wear trousers, wear a skirt instead (or vice versa).

- Carry a handbag, not a carry-all (or vice versa).

- If you generally wear make-up then go fresh faced.

- Get the bus instead of taking the car, or take the car instead of the train.

- Buy tea if you usually buy coffee on the way into work.

- Take the stairs rather than using the lift.

- If you tend to make tea then use herbal tea or make coffee instead.

- If you normally go out to lunch, buy a sandwich to eat at your desk or bring in a packed lunch.

- If you call your friends in the afternoon, call them in the morning instead.

- Leave work later or earlier than you normally do.

- Take a different route home.

- Eat out if you usually eat in, or cook something that you have never had before, or get a friend to cook.

- Watch television if you normally read, or read if you usually watch television.

- Call your parents today instead of (routinely) on Friday.

- Do the weekly shopping late in the evening instead of (routinely) on Saturday morning.

- Apply moisturiser if you don't do so normally and then turn off the light.

Any of the above activities could make you look at your day completely differently. You may want to make such changes permanently, or decide to go back to normal.

Be different, refreshing and inspiring.

JUST MAKE UP WHAT YOU WANT

Today you have permission to daydream about anything you want to. You can think about all the things you wish for and all the things you dream about.

Today is total release from the real world. You can wish for anything you want and live in your own personal dream world.

You must, of course, have some real fun at the start by writing down ten wishes or dreams. They must be totally personal and can be very selfish, but they must be things that are currently in your head, or things that you sometimes mull over in your mind during the day. Your dreams and wishes should be your real dreams and wishes. Go for it! You may, for instance, want to:

- Sing with Frank Sinatra/Elvis Presley.

- Fly to the moon.

- Fly around the world in a hot-air balloon.

- Be 6 feet tall.

- Have an IQ of 200.

- Rule the world.

Once you have made the list, just sit back and enjoy it. Imagine yourself ruling the world – shortly after winning *Mastermind*. Tickets to the moon in your back pocket and the smell of the greasepaint and roar of the crowd still fresh in your mind from last night's concert, with Elvis as backing. Waiting to hear from the palace for an appointment to measure up for your crown. Feels good, doesn't it, and I bet you have at least a smile on your face if you haven't laughed out loud.

It's great – in your mind you can be and do anything you want to do. So go ahead, dream on and wish away.

Now that you have got into the swing of it you can get on with your normal day and transform it into the most amazing day you have ever had – a 'day-dream'. Everything you do today is the stuff that dreams are made of.

Leave your palace early in the morning to travel to the *Mastermind* studios. Help some university students on their way with their dissertations.

Give Elvis some hints and tips on being successful as a pop star. Meet up with some old friends for lunch and decide to take the whole afternoon off in order to shop for everything you have ever wanted but simply haven't had the time to buy. When you have picked up the children from school you will be going to see Mickey Mouse, who has called to say that he has a spare hour or so and asked to come and entertain the children while you prepare the sumptuous evening meal. After having the meal the children say they want to go to bed as they are tired and you and your partner fly off to the coast in the hot-air balloon to see the sun set. Once you return you can pay the babysitter and go to bed – to awake to a breakfast of fresh fruit salad in a champagne juice with lightly poached eggs on light French toast. Get the picture?

You see, I have everything and anything I want, every day of my life. I just dream for 5 minutes and there it all is – it doesn't cost a penny and it feels sooooooo good.

'Dreamers' and 'people who wish their life away' are

sometimes considered to be negative, as if they have no real aim in life or cannot come to terms with what is real. If you know that you are dreaming or wishing, and you can return to the real world happy and refreshed, having had a little entertainment and excitement, then I think that you and other dreamers and wishers are probably the only people who have a real idea of what is going on. They are aware of the real world and of their own very personal world – the world of their own minds. And everyone knows that if you know your own mind, you are strong and can do anything.

Well done, you now have a crystal-clear picture of where you are going and how good it feels.

You have the confidence of youth and the wisdom of age. You are totally sorted and empowered.

PART 3

Your Soul

9

Stay Young, Energised and Spiritualised Detox

There is a balance in our lives that may be described as 'mind, body and spirit' or 'physical, emotional and energetic'. However it is termed, it is completely essential that we look at every dimension of our life in order to get the best out of it. If we eat well to stay young, and if we think well enough to stop negative thoughts from keeping us young and detoxed, then we also need some support structures that we can call on when the programme reveals some further questions or doubts.

Many people have a religion or a belief structure. This section is in no way meant to replace or change those religious beliefs. On the contrary, it should complement them and add to them in an amusing, interesting and enlightening way – hopefully in a way you haven't thought of before and one that helps the Stay Young Detox work wonderfully for you.

We will look at several ways to enhance and empower you and your life, and to detox to stay young at heart. Whichever way you choose, they are each designed to energise, fulfil and expand – to give you confidence in yourself so that you will feel youthful and daring again.

Each of these methods will be complementary to your

current life – whether it enhances what you already believe, or adds to a life with no belief structure. It will also be complementary because it will give you more ways to empower yourself and enable you to do anything you want to do.

THE ENERGY OR SPIRIT

Have you ever had the experience of feeling that someone is not well and finding out that they are, indeed, not well when you call them? Have you ever thought of someone for the first time in ages shortly before they telephoned you? Have you ever said anything bad about someone when they were standing right behind you, when you were sure they had left the building? Have you ever concentrated very hard on something being how you want it to be and it came true? Have you ever asked someone to guess what choice you made and they guessed correctly, despite the fact that they knew nothing about the subject? Have you ever known categorically that someone or something wasn't right and then were proved correct? All this is your use of energy. It involves tuning in to energy levels and signs and then making them work for you. Energy can be used in many ways and not least by you. From this point on, you can become more familiar with your own energy and look at ways to use it and benefit from it.

Complementary practitioners often talk about energy work, and many people talk about the flow of energy. It isn't always clear what they mean. People frequently say that their energy is low or that a lack of energy is a problem for them. Some people have 'bad energy' and some are 'high in energy'. Some people are nice to be around, even if they are not saying anything, while others can make a room feel dark just by being in it. Practitioners may talk about blocked energy and some people play with and use their energy to get what they wish for and take themselves to a place where they want to be.

Whatever your view of the source of energy – spiritual or very physical – there is no doubt that we could all do with good energy levels. This section of the Stay Young Detox looks at energy on all levels and of every type. You will be able to use this energy to confound people who have put you down to being over the hill or stuck in your ways. You will amaze yourself when you can do things you had decided were now beyond your means. Quite simply, you will be harnessing your energy.

There are many types of energy:

- The Indian life force is prana.

- The Chinese life force, or energy flow, is chi, qi or ki, which can be divided into male and female, or yang and yin respectively.

- Native Americans have Mother Earth and Father Sky.

- Reiki healers have the Universal Life Force.

Energy can also be found in many forms, including chakras, meridians and energy channels, or simply free flow that we can harness for use and then release.

There is much, much more than we can consider here, but we need to start somewhere and here is as good a place as any.

For this part of the 9 steps to the Stay Young Detox, you should choose any of the following to support your every step of the programme. You can choose one and use it to empower you from day 1 to day 18, or opt for a different source for yourself every day of the 18 days. You could use several sources or concentrate on just one – the choice is yours. Some of the sources are more conventional than others, and some are more unusual, but they are all interesting and definitely effective and honourable.

Your Sources of Empowerment

Feng shui	Capture the chi and get it to flow freely around your home for prosperity, health and relationship success.
Animal medicine	Choose your favourite animal, or see what visits the garden, look up the medicine associated with it and see what message it has for you. Alternatively, choose the animal medicine you need and imagine your new pet tiger at your heel.
Aromatherapy	Get to the essence of your needs by choosing the oil for detox or for rejuvenation.
Crystal healing	Every stone can be turned. Every quality can be provided. Use crystals to sparkle and radiate.
Yoga	Breathe life into your body and revitalise your mind. Stretch the very corners of your being and spring back with youth.
Chakra energy	Calm yourself down or speed yourself up by using your own energy to the best advantage.

Once you've used it, close it down, put it away and save it for another day. Total empowerment.

Space clearing — Clear out old baggage, divest yourself of the past and move forwards with renewed vigour. Clear the clutter and cleanse the space.

FENG SHUI

For this programme you could decide that you are going to look at ways of clearing the rooms in your home so that the chi will flow freely and support you in your endeavours. Get the best from your surroundings and free flow your positive energy.

The Chinese art of placement, or feng shui, has become increasingly popular in the West. Feng shui is about harnessing energy and getting it to flow freely through your life and your home or workplace. Wherever we exist there is chi, the energy flow. If we block off a door or move a window to an inconvenient spot, we could disrupt or decrease the potential flow of good energy in our lives. If we live in a strange place or in a place affected by extreme circumstances, we could be missing out on or positively discouraging the flow of good energy in our lives. Feng shui and its application will optimise the flow of good energy into your life, and the flow of bad energy away from you or out of your life.

Why not design our homes so that we bring health, wealth and happiness into our lives, as well as a patterned border and bunk beds in the children's room for extra storage? We spend huge amounts of our incomes on our homes and dwellings, and most people living in the West spend a great deal of time making their day-to-day lives more enjoyable. We strive to make the most of our lives and do the best we can. We do all this by following simple rules of existence that have been passed down from generation to generation, and we don't give it a second thought. We choose colours we like, we choose houses by the look of them from the driveway, we rebuild to knock rooms together or extend into open space. We design our gardens for the optimum look and minimum effort, and we search the antique shops to find the ultimate doorstop.

There are many other cultures that follow their own sets of rules and operate in much the same way. Some of these cultures attach a little more importance to their surroundings and the effects that they have on them than others. People in Tibet and Vietnam follow *Phong Thuy*; in the Philippines, Indonesia and Thailand they follow *Hong Sui* and in Japan, Hawaii and India they believe in *Vaastu Shastra*.

The Chinese use the rules and science of feng shui (pronounced fung shway, or fung shoy), much of which has been introduced throughout the world due to interest from Western cultures. Its popularity is due to our increasing desire to get the best out of our homes and, more importantly, to become happier, healthier and wealthier individuals. It seems to be entirely British that we shouldn't admit to wanting to make money, be successful and become prosperous. Feng shui allows this and supports the desire to make the most of what we have got.

Feng Shui is a philosophy, of Chinese origin, which maintains that the configurations of the earth shape the affairs of the people that live among them.

Derek Walters

The two characters feng and shui literally mean wind and water, and this really denotes the fact that feng shui is concerned with earthly and not spiritual influences. Feng shui is not a religion or an art, but a science. There are strict rules of application and along with the overall philosophy there are numerous tools, techniques and exercises to be used when introducing feng shui principles into your life.

Simply put, feng shui is about getting all the positive energy available to you into your life, keeping it there, using it to its optimum and then allowing all negative energy a free route out of your life. Keeping up a constant flow of good energy without any blockages will bring health, wealth and prosperity – something we could all do with more of.

There are many schools of feng shui, and to dictate the school you should follow would be arrogant of me, but there are also many books and magazines that you can read in order to find out the basics.

The best way to ensure that you are following feng shui principles is to get a consultation done. These can be very expensive, but if you find a fully qualified practitioner who has studied for many years rather than just done a few weekend courses (*see Resources, page 220*), you will find that the results of the consultation will undoubtedly be worth the initial outlay.

While you are deciding how to introduce feng shui into

your life there are some simple tools that you can use which can start you on your journey.

As stated earlier, feng shui has a lot to do with the flow of energy. In order for energy to flow it needs to have all blockages or obstacles removed. Anything that would shut it off, or redirect it or prevent it from entering every aspect of your home should be rectified. In the same way, anything that speeds up the energy or results in too much energy should be carefully looked at so that a balanced flow is maintained.

Stand outside your home on the street and face your front door. Imagine that you are the positive energy. Look around you and begin to judge if there is anything that is preventing easy access to your home. Is there a tree across your front door? Is your front door old and dirty? Is the drive long and funnel-like so that too much energy speeds up towards the door and overpowers it, or is the path just long enough for the energy to arrive at the door ready for entry?

Does the front door work, or does it stick (get that fixed). Does your hallway lead you through the house, or is there a wall in the way that blocks the flow? Is there a door you never use or that is blocked by a piece of furniture? If there is, clear the blockage and open the door to let the energy flow in. Have you got mirrors facing each other? As a rule they just bounce energy backwards and forwards, which is disruptive and interferes with the flow; move them so that they don't reflect each other but reflect the energy out into the house and encourage its path. Hang all doors so that they open into the rooms and not back out into the hall or corridor, so that when you approach a room you naturally flow into it. Check that the back door is not blocked and opens outwards so that all energy, once it has passed through the house and been used, can exit freely. Check, however, that the front door is not in line with the back door, as this arrangement will make energy entering your home then zoom straight out of the back of your property before it gets to circulate its beneficial properties.

Once you have completed your journey through the house you will be more aware of your home dynamics and may wish to make some changes to get the optimum flow. You have now completed some basic steps to implementing feng shui into your life. You have detoxed the negative energy and promoted the positive energy. Well done.

ANIMAL MEDICINE

Use the wildlife around you and the animals that creep into your thoughts to empower your every move. Listen to what they are telling you and act accordingly – remember, animals don't tell lies and they have no hidden agendas.

Animals have their own life force. We know that spending time with animals can have therapeutic benefits. Animals are used in hospitals and homes to relax and inspire patients or residents, and they are used in therapy to interact at an honest level. Their energy is comforting and calming. If you couple this energy with their individual characteristics, you will have different types of spirit and/or energy. This is the essence of animal medicine. You find out about yourself through the animal energy that visits you or you think about or summon into your life.

Animal medicine is used in Native American culture and it has nothing to do with taking a substance internally by spoon or pill. It can be used for inspiration, confidence, support and guidance. It can act like a friend and can help you through the more difficult challenges you face. It can also be lighthearted or enable you to be lighthearted and frivolous. Indeed, this medicine can be taken for everything. You can choose what you take and when you take it, and you can use it just whenever you want to.

I have included animal medicine in the Stay Young Detox programme because of its flexibility. Staying young, as we have discussed, is as much a state of mind as it is a physical condition.

We may feel that we are getting older when we are faced with something that we cannot deal with easily. We label lack of confidence, lack of knowledge, confusion, inability to cope, and so on, under the umbrella phrase of 'I'm getting old', or we put it down to 'That terminal condition called life'.

What we can do is to find a tool that gives us back all the things we think we have lost through ageing, or even gives us something for the first time, the lack of which we have been able to blame on ageing.

Animal medicine is just such a tool. Animal medicine treats anything and everything exactly when you want it to. It visits when least expected and can be called upon as and when you need it. You are probably already using it in one way or another – or at least it is probably already in your life without your knowing it.

Before I describe how animal medicine works I should just take a few words to explain that it is not a religion or a cult. It is simply a way of empowering your life. It can enhance your belief system and become a belief system. If none of this appeals, just read about it and see how interesting the interpretations of the animals are and how they could compare with some people you know.

Animals do not stand on ceremony; they do not tell you what you want to hear; they do not lie; and they do not make you feel guilty. Animals just are. They spend their lives surviving and that is their main agenda. Most animals are prey to other animals, so surviving is big on their 'to do' list. We could actually learn a lot from them, and we can certainly benefit from their 'medicine'.

Wild animals live on the Earth quite freely, and they find ways to survive. When we domesticate them for our own pleasure and use, they lose some of their independence but none of their 'animal instincts'. Pet cats will still bring in shrews, mice and birds despite having a bowlful of food served to them on a regular basis. Horses at a riding stables will shy away or kick out if you approach their blind spot. They have an innate survival instinct.

Every animal has a certain set of qualities, and every animal can help us in totally different ways. Every animal can be called upon, and every animal is likely to have visited you at some time in your life. If you have pets you are likely to have been receiving animal medicine all along! What is more soothing than to hold an animal on your lap when you are stressed or tired? What is funnier than watching animals play at fighting and biffing each other with their paws? What is more mesmerising than watching fish in a tank swimming without a care in the world?

I have chosen a few of the more common animals for

you to start with, but every animal has its own medicine. You can start to see that you can get everything you want from animal medicine, and animal medicine will visit you just whenever you least expect it. Here are the animals and advice on some of the ways you can use them to empower you to have the confidence of youth.

The prescription

How do we take animal medicine? It really is incredibly simple. If you need anything, like confidence or support, or any of the qualities described above, then you can just think of the animal that has those qualities. If you imagine the animal and see it moving in your mind's eye, you are taking the medicine and benefiting from everything the animal can give you.

As an example, you might decide that before going on a hot date you could do with some help or confidence. Now, reading about cats we see that they are magical and mysterious, and that they hunt at night and sleep curled up during the day. They remain wary of danger and can look after themselves quite capably and independently. How wonderfully exotic! You can learn from them the glamour of having a confident night out, but with the care and caution that befits a first night. Start to take cat medicine and see your confidence and demeanour develop.

As you are getting ready, imagine the purring of the contented cat mixed with the fun and playfulness of a kitten and the wisdom and security of the night hunter. Absolutely nothing can faze you and nothing can prevent you from having a wonderful time.

Cat medicine applies to both male and female. Think

of the bigger cats – the puma, the lynx – and think of witches' mysterious black cats. Male or female, choose your cat of choice and drink its medicine.

Similarly, you may feel that something is not quite right, and that you are not getting to the bottom of something. If you are feeling not so flushed with the brashness of youth, you may not want to stride in and accuse someone of something that you think could be going on – or not going on. Think owl medicine. Imagine yourself away from the situation, flying above it with your penetrating night vision. Imagine your owl hooting as your deep notes resonate through to find the truth. You can see everything clearly and you can see through everything. Owl medicine will give you the wisdom you need to deal with the situation. You will be able to see what is true and confront the situation or people and get things sorted.

Taking the medicine is not something you have to do before a situation. The beauty of animal medicine is that it can happen anywhere, any time. In a meeting, if your job description is being discussed or if there is change in the company, just imagine a crow on a perch behind you, sharing your situation. Crows see universal law and justice and help with change. Bring in the crow and see change happen for the better.

Coyote medicine is my personal favourite. When I get a little too serious or bogged down by deadlines, or nervous about demonstrations or public speaking, I stroke my pet coyote that hangs out by my right leg. He will often wander away but just when I need the support, he comes straight back to heel, like a faithful but light-hearted dog, looking after me. With coyote medicine I can balance just about anything.

Other people can take this medicine and you can send this medicine to others. If you have children at college and it is exam time, or if your friends are travelling around the world and you are worried about them, think of an appropriate animal and send them the medicine. They will receive it. In the same way, if an animal visits you, for instance if you open your curtains one morning and there are birds on your lawn, look up their medicine and see what the day holds. If you are out walking and a horse rides by, what are you being told? What is being sent to you to help you? If you see a mouse in the corner of an alleyway while sitting in a traffic jam, are you looking at the details or are you getting bogged down in the detail and not seeing the wood for the trees?

The animals

Spider

Spider medicine is that of creation. It is about weaving your web and creating your own fate or destiny. Spider medicine can be used to weave yourself into or out of a situation; it is about your future. If you have the ability to weave, then you have the ability to create anything you want. Just as with a spider's web, what you 'weave' can be re-created or expanded or reduced. It can entrap, and feed and nourish, or it can protect and encase. With spider medicine you can create your own future.

Horse

Horse medicine is about travel and freedom. Horses gave

people the ability to leave their immediate surroundings and to visit new, uncharted territory. Horses are work animals, they take people from a to b; they take goods to market; and they pull carts and carriages. Horses are strong and poweful, and horse medicine shows you your life in terms of travel, broadening horizons and moving on. It is about what journey you are on in your life and how to move in a new direction, to feel freedom and to have the power to move on.

Ant

People often find the idea of ant medicine very humorous. The idea that something as small as an ant can have any effect on our lives seems strange. But think of the power of the small ant that often carries weights many times its own body size. Ants are always with other ants; if you ever see them they are working away at feeding the queen ant. They have the patience to work for others, and to do what is needed until their rewards come, little by little. Ant medicine teaches us that if we work hard and methodically, 'everything will come to those who wait'. Ants are industrious; you never see an ant relaxing, for they are always doing something. What they do is never random, but it always has a purpose. Hard work pays off: this is the medicine of the ant.

Wolf

Wolf medicine is intelligent medicine. Like dogs, wolves are faithful animals. They have families and stay with them. They mate for life. They run with the pack and they hunt alone. Wolves have a very strict code of conduct within their family. They have a strict pecking order and they are very loyal.

Wolves guard their families with great protection. They are intelligent and make decisions based on the levels of danger they face. We are led to believe that wolves are dangerous, but for them attack is always the last resort. Wolves look at all the options and then take the least dangerous route forwards. They remain in control, and take decisions and make moves that enable them to feel safe when getting to where they want to be. Wolf medicine guards and protects, enabling you to make the moves you wish safely and intelligently.

Owl

Owl medicine is about seeing the truth. It is about seeing deception for what it is and avoiding it. Owls hunt at night. They have night vision, and they are more seeing than we are. The 'wise old owl' will always see the truth in any situation. It is for this reason that owl medicine is about knowledge and wisdom, for the owl can see when we cannot, and it can see even when it is dark and things are hidden to the normal eye; owls can see the truth however it is disguised. Owl medicine will enable you to see the truth and move forwards with confidence, knowing that you have all the facts.

Dolphin

Many people travel long distances just for the chance to swim with dolphins. Dolphins represent freedom and nature, laughter and joy. After having swum with dolphins, people talk of being filled with feelings of inner peace, joy and relaxation which are so powerful that they change their perception of their own lives. 'Until I swam with dolphins I didn't fully appreciate the wonder of nature', is not an uncommon reaction. They have the ability – being mammals – to hold their breath and swim with a wonderful rhythm, using the air to its full capacity.

Swimming with dolphins takes us to a place of contentment, freedom, joy and peace, to a dreamlike state where everything is in proportion and nothing really matters. It's a truly spiritual and energetic experience. Think of dolphins and breathe in new life and joy and have some fun. Let go and move forwards with confidence, feeling that you have the breath of life.

Bat

Some people don't really like this little creature of the night. Its depiction as the screeching monster that flies at you in the depths of darkness seems to signify fear and terror. Bat medicine is about facing your fears. It's about doing what needs to be done and moving on. Bat medicine can often mean the end of one thing and the beginning of another – the darkness before the dawn. It can have connections with death, but death does not always mean sadness. The death of something also means the birth of something new or new beginnings. Bat medicine asks you to face the truth and perhaps the fear, to confront it and then to move forwards. Bats signify new starts with wisdom and knowing. There's nothing evil about them at all!

Deer

Deer medicine is about caring, compassion and gentleness. Think of a deer and you simultaneously go soft and cuddly. Think of the phrase 'doe eyes', and you imagine large, wide, innocent and sweet eyes. Think of deer in a park and you will know that one small crack of a twig will send them off at speed to a place of safety. They are perceptive, and know that they should look after themselves to protect themselves. Deer medicine is about exactly this; taking care of yourself, taking time to see that you are looked after and caring for yourself. If you look after yourself and others with utmost care you will be repaid. This is the time to reflect and relax, not to forge forwards beating your brow. Deer medicine is about gentleness and calm.

Bear

Big huggy bears have the power and ability to kill at one move. They know when to strike and when to retreat. Bears do not hibernate totally, but they do become reclusive as they are rearing their cubs for many months. They disappear and re-emerge in the spring with new cubs and new life. They eat honey, a sweet substance that you would, perhaps, associate more readily with a smaller, more frivolous animal, but bear medicine is about looking deep inside ourselves to find the inner power. Once this is found, we can experience the sweet taste of life.

Bears signify power, physical strength and inner strength. Go forwards with a bear at your side and you can be safe in the knowledge that your beliefs are based on a great deal of thought and introspection and topped with the sweet taste of honeyed success.

Dog

Dogs are man's best friend. They serve their master and are loyal to the end. Dog medicine is about loyalty to others and to yourself. No matter how badly a dog is treated it will still return to serve. If it is shown a little care, it will remain a best friend and do everything you ask of it. Show it bad habits that you approve of, and it will copy them. Dog medicine tells you to look at your habits: are you serving your friends and family loyally and with care, or have you got into bad habits that they are putting up with and going along with because they love you? Are you being true to yourself, or are you letting your bad habits get the best of you? Look at your life, be true to your core values and be your own best friend, not just everybody else's.

Dragon-fly

The dragon-fly is amazingly coloured and the light changes its iridescence with every angle of flight. It flies during the day and the light dances on its wings and shows its true colours. It has two pairs of wings, but can adapt and fly with only one. Its colours transform and change. Dragon-fly medicine is about change and adaptability. If a dragon-fly flies into your thoughts or you see one in your garden, think about whether you are being flexible. Are you able to change and adapt, or are you set in your habits and not able to change? Change brings opportunity and new beginnings.

Squirrel

Squirrels hoard and collect for the winter months ahead. They collect and store. They have things put by to serve them later, and they have stocks or reserves that they can call upon. Squirrel medicine is about being prepared for anything, so that nothing will faze you or throw you out of step. The downside of squirrel medicine is being too prepared and having too much hoarded, so that there is clutter preventing you from reacting, responding or even just moving forwards.

Squirrels get the balance right. If squirrel medicine is what you need it is telling you that if you do not need or use something, if you cannot see a valuable use for it in the future, then do not hoard. Clear the clutter back to your needs and requirements. Anything surplus to this can go or be given back. You are then in balance, prepared but not stagnating. You have the resources but no restrictions. You will be able to deal with anything life throws at you without getting confused and bogged down with the unnecessary.

Coyote

As mentioned before, coyote medicine is my favourite – moreover, it is the medicine that I am always told I should take more of. Once when I was doing a demonstration massage treatment, a lady said to me that she could see animal guides, and that throughout the treatment my coyote was at my heels looking out for me. I love this image and the thought of the support it gives me, so now when I work with clients I just say a silent hello to my coyote!

Coyotes teach you about yourself. They are about learning and they are about lightening up and having fun. The coyote is mischievous and has the ability to trick others and also itself. Coyote medicine is about playing the fool and having fun and not taking things too seriously. It is about making sure you are not fooling yourself by ignoring the obvious, and it is about the balance between the fun in life and the knowing.

Whale

Whales are the biggest mammals, and they swim deep and communicate with sound and song. We don't often see whales. We go in search of them, and then wait hours to get a glimpse of this invisible creature. When a whale thrusts itself out of the water, either with its strong, powerful tail-fin or by throwing its whole body upwards and forwards, we can begin to see the magic. Keeping yourself hidden and your talents to yourself can mean that you become lost in your own deep, dark world. Sharing your creativity and developing your thoughts will bring you out into the world to share your creativity and let it grow. Whale medicine tells us that we should use our creativity and let others benefit from it – burst out and let it expand other people's lives as well as your own.

Eagle

Eagles are powerful birds, flying high above, kings of all they survey, and swooping down on their prey once they have got the best view. Eagle medicine is about seeing all the facts, knowing the truth and then using this to your best advantage. It is about not staying Earth-bound and only seeing things from one level. Eagle medicine tells us to soar high, find new perspectives and enjoy the flight. Go to a new level and check the view. Everything will look much clearer from your new perspective.

Snake

The snake is like the bat, and some people only see its traditional serpent aspect – the poisonous venom and the cold, slippery nature. Snake medicine is nothing like this; it is about rebirth. The snake sheds its skin and is reborn. It therefore has many lives and with this comes much wisdom. The snake has knowledge: it is used in the symbol for Western medicine to show healing. It represents transition, travel from one stage to another, for snakes react and respond at speed, seeing danger and moving fleetingly. Snake medicine is relevant to rapid change, rebirth and wisdom. Like the serpent, the snake is hypnotic and enchanting and will hold you in its spell.

Swan

Swans are very feminine. Swan medicine is about grace, but remember the swan's legs, which work powerfully under the water's surface to create the scene of calm and serenity. Swan medicine is about the beauty of the female, and her intuition and power. It will allow you to finally see what you already know but have been denying. I am often told to look at swan medicine as I try to be more intuitive with my clients. If you think about a friend whom you haven't seen for ages, or if you talk to a colleague and something seems wrong – really talk to them. If you say you think they are not their normal self, you will find that they will be able to share their burdens with someone who has recognised their difficulty and their call for help.

Rabbit

We talk about rabbits caught in the headlights when describing someone who is in a state of abject fear. Rabbit medicine is about recognising our own fears and getting them into a place where we can deal with them. Running scared gets us nowhere. We must work out what we are afraid of, find the solution and move forwards safely and without restriction. Being afraid means that we may end up never leaving the house for fear of what *might happen*. If we can address our fears we will find that it will never happen and will be free to live our lives. Don't worry unnecessarily. Don't try to control what may never actually happen. Rabbit medicine is about confronting fear, putting it into perspective and moving on.

Butterfly

Butterflies are about transformation. Butterfly medicine is about the continuing cycle of never-ending transformation. How am I changing? Am I developing? Have I moved on? Have I moved up? Am I developing in the way I want to? Do I want change? Butterfly medicine allows you to check in with these questions about your life, and then lets you change into something you want to be. It permits you to make the right decision so that you can achieve what you desire. The beautiful butterfly will fly upwards and show its new colours; it tells us that only with change can we grow, and that change makes us more beautiful.

Fox

The cunning fox can get to where it wants to be – the best vantage point or the position of safety – without ever being seen. We see foxes in our gardens, always just passing through, slinking away into the hedge or under the shed. They play and hypnotise with their graceful actions while moving in for the kill of their prey. Foxes watch every move; they see the patterns and know when to strike. Fox medicine will enable you to see the moves that others around you make, so that you will be able to join in or move away at exactly the right times. The art of camouflage is the art of the fox. It's about cunning, about knowing when to use its sly power and when to retreat into the hedgerow, never to be seen again. Fox medicine teaches us to retreat, see a situation and then blend into the solution. Cunningness and slyness will protect and serve you with this medicine.

Crow

Crow medicine is secret and magical, creative and spiritual. The crow is about balance, natural laws, the laws of the jungle and the laws of respect for others, and about humanity and integrity. Crow medicine helps us to seek out that which is right and to follow it. Crows bring magical change. They are black as night and signify the new dawn. Crows remind us that there is magic in everything and everything is magical. Seeing crows in your day will mean that magical change is just around the corner.

Cat

Cats are independent; they have an air of mystery and despite being very domesticated, they have an image of being very aloof. Black cats have the magical aspect of the spirit world. A black cat crossing your path is meant to signify good luck, or that you are being asked to be aware of what is going on around you. Cats have 9 lives and they have curiosity – that doesn't often kill them! The cat is the chosen pet of the witch – riding high on the broomstick. When we keep cats as pets we tend to call them in at night and make them comfortable in a basket or bed, but the cat is, in fact, a night animal, prowling and catching animals to eat and to bring to its owners as gifts. Cats are mysterious and magical, and if cat medicine is in your life you should be prepared for the magical mystery tour you are about to go on.

Mouse

Watch a mouse and see it examine every detail. It picks things up, sniffs and nibbles, and only when things are up to muster are they allowed out of the grips of mouse medicine. Mouse medicine is in the detail, every last detail, in fact. They say that the devil is in the detail. If this is so, the mouse will never fall prey to the devil, since it checks and examines everything to see if it is all right before progressing. Mouse medicine makes us take a second look; it makes us check that we are not missing the obvious, so that we can escape unhurt. It makes us check the small print. Mouse medicine can also tell us that we are getting too bogged down in the detail and that we should free our minds and look at the bigger picture. Mouse medicine is essentially detail – check if there is enough or too much in your life and take the medicine.

Animal medicine is so versatile and so much fun. Use it and you can be just whoever you want to be, do just whatever takes your fancy or whatever you need to do. Animal medicine is empowering and will keep you young forever. Animals do not work with your age; they work with your being.

AROMATHERAPY AND ESSENTIAL OILS

Aromatherapy is the use of essential oils extracted from flowers and plants for the medicinal healing of mind, body and spirit.

Most people still think that aromatherapy is simply a massage using scented oils. This could not be further from the truth. The strength and potency of essential oils is still not fully appreciated, but if you have ever experienced a true aromatherapy treatment you will understand just how valuable they can be in our lives.

Essential oils are administered in many ways: massage, aromatherapy, compresses, inhalations, local application, bathing and burning, to name just a few. Whichever way you experience them you should be aware that in the right doses they are incredibly effective, but in the wrong doses or applications they can be correspondingly dangerous and potentially damaging. I personally know this fact only too well. When I was first introduced to these amazing oils I remember applying basil oil directly to my wrists, just as you would apply perfume, in order to carry the smell with me. The resulting circular burn on both wrists soon proved to me that these were no ordinary fragrant oils.

There is absolutely nothing new in essential oils or the use of plants in healing. Some of the most potent and dangerous drugs are derived purely from plant extracts – think of opium from the poppy plant, cocaine from the coca plant and digitalis, the heart drug, from the foxglove plant. This is an illustration of just how effective essential oils can be.

Having said all that I don't for one minute want to stop anybody from benefiting from the fabulous qualities of essential oils and aromatherapy treatments. From the history of aromatherapy and the use of plants in natural medicine it is obvious that this is definitely not a new therapy. In fact, it could be deemed to be one of the more ancient therapies still available to us today.

Oils have been used for embalming and preparing bodies for the afterworld from as early as 3000 BC. Records of the Incas of Peru, Mapuche healers of Chile and the ancient Greeks and Romans, and medieval documents, all show evidence that herbal mixes and scented oils were used as an integral part of their medicine chests. As we get nearer to the present day we can again see that in the 18th and 19th centuries, plant extracts played a crucial role in the development of powerful and effective drugs. Today, these drugs are becoming increasingly available to the general public.

We will now look at just how fabulous essential oils can be if used correctly and in the right quantities, and how beneficial they can be for the Stay Young Detox programme.

You should start by asking yourself some key questions, which will help you get the best out of your oils:

- What effect do I want?

- What format do I want to try?

- What amounts should I be using?

Once you have answered these questions you can take the next steps to enjoying the amazing effects of your chosen oils and treatment.

What effect do I want?

Here is a list (by no means definitive) of oils that I recommend as extremely beneficial to the Stay Young Detox programme. You can see from this that almost every aspect of your life can be addressed with the use of essential oils and aromatherapy. Mind, body and spirit can be worked on separately or at the same time. Specific illnesses or emotions can be addressed, and you can even change your state of mind. There really is nothing that essential oils cannot help with, work on or eliminate.

Study this list to see what each oil can do. You may decide that it provides enough information; if an effect you require is not listed you can consult other books in a library or bookshop to work out which oil or blend you need.

Geranium

This is a generally uplifting and balancing oil. If you need calm, geranium is an oil you should have in your first-aid kit. It is also good for happiness, harmony, balance, inner strength, liberation, regeneration and tranquillity.

Grapefruit

This refreshing citrus oil is clean smelling and crisp. It has many properties valuable to the Stay Young Detox: diuretic, anti-cellulite, balancing, energising, liberating, revitalising and very uplifting. It may help to boost self-awareness, confidence and positive thinking.

Basil

I used to burn this oil together with ginger when I first went into business, and found it very empowering and positive. It is anti-cellulite, energising, and good for positive thinking. Remember that the herb is just as good to eat.

Frankincense

Often thought of as a religious oil, this is indeed a very spiritual oil; it is also very uplifting. It is assuring, cleansing and inspirational, and can help with emotional stability, empowerment and wisdom.

Juniper

This is very detoxing and cleansing. It is a very strong diuretic, good for fighting cellulite, cleansing and energising, and can be used to enhance a positive mind, self-worth, vitality and wisdom. Juniper is a key detox oil to own.

Lavender

This is one of the safest oils to use. It is balancing both physically and emotionally, gives inner peace, and is liberating, regenerative and also very relaxing and calming.

Rosemary

You couldn't ask much more from an oil. Rosemary is totally balancing and a good, all-round player. It is excellent for fighting cellulite, self-awareness, centring, energising and helping to gain a positive mind.

Ginger

This is warming, assuring and centring, and gives confidence, feelings of being in control and happiness. Sounds like a total cure-all! It is, perhaps, most appropriate in the winter months, but still has the same effects all year round. Eat the ginger root on top of your breakfast yoghurt or grated on to salads.

Fennel

Eat the fennel bulb or use the oil. Both are diuretic, revitalising and great for digestion, helping the large intestine and acting as an antiseptic for the gut.

Pine

This is good for cleansing, being in control and energising. It is no coincidence that cleaning products are often fragranced with pine essence. Cleansing and energising are definitely results we can benefit from on the Stay Young Detox programme.

Ylang ylang

Some find this oil too flowery, but think in terms of exotic island holidays and you cannot fail to benefit from the uplifting and sensual properties of this oil. Use it to feel awakened, confident and uplifted.

Eucalyptus

Apart from having a fresh, clean perfume, eucalyptus is wonderfully balancing, energising and regenerating. It is no surprise that the eucalyptus tree is one of the fastest growing and strongest trees around, and the Australians swear by its medicinal regenerative properties.

Rose otto

Like ylang ylang, rose otto is wonderfully flowery and

feminine. It is great for skin care, revitalising and balancing, and generates feelings of happiness, inner peace, inspiration, regeneration and all-round knowing.

Lemon

The qualities of this essential oil include: diuretic, anti-cellulite, energising, revitalising, good for self-awareness, cleansing, inspirational, helps with positive thinking, revitalising, anti-acid and really easy to get hold of. Mix it with grapefruit and ginger in a burner and you'll find that the smell alone is a total tonic.

Pre-prepared blend or single oils?

The only comparison that can be drawn between essential oils for medicinal use and perfume oils for fragrances is that both need to be blended carefully to ensure that they still remain effective and pleasant to the nose. Simply looking at the list above and ticking off the oils with the effects that you wish to experience is one thing. Blending them together with no experience or knowledge can result in nothing more than a nasty-smelling mixture.

Once you have chosen your oils you should make a further decision – do you want to use pre-prepared blends or mix the oils yourself?

If you are buying or using your own essential oils I recommend that you keep it really simple. Use one or perhaps two oils at any one time. This will ensure that you will be able to tell which oil is working for you, and that your blends will smell nice.

There is a lot to be said for using pre-prepared blends.

It is not cheating – it is in fact probably much more beneficial. Not only has someone done the work for you; they have also used their skill and knowledge to achieve a blend that works therapeutically and still smells wonderfully good. Home blending can result in a strange concoction that will never leave the bathroom shelf! Home blending can also reduce the effectiveness of the oils. You may not be able to buy the exact combination you are after, but this could be because such a combination simply doesn't work either therapeutically or fragrantly. Just like in chemistry, mixing substances can result in more than you bargained for, or in the case of aromatherapy – less than you bargained for. If you don't understand the exact constituents of the oils you could be cancelling out some of their effects if you mix them together.

If you buy a blend you are guaranteed that all the oils in the mix work well together and are possibly more effective together. Pre-prepared blends can be a little expensive but they are likely to have years of experience and knowledge behind them.

A pointer when buying blends is an oil's colour. Natural oils and carrier or base oils are neutral in colour, or vary from clear to deep brown, or green like olive oil. Very few natural oils have pigment that could be termed a colour. Blue chamomile is one exception as it is dark blue, and bergamot is deep orange, but certainly none of them is purple, red or pink! When buying blends, make sure they are totally natural.

What format do I want to try?

This is where the fun starts. There are so many ways to enjoy and benefit from essential oils that you won't know exactly where to start! Here are some suggestions to help you make a decision.

Professional aromatherapy massage

This is one of my favourite ways to experience aromatherapy. You will experience a treatment, usually lasting an hour, where the therapist will work over your whole body. The massage strokes are designed to stimulate the circulation and warm the body. The skin then absorbs the essential oil, which then travels into the blood and lymph system to have its effect throughout the body. It is best not to shower after a treatment to enable the essential oils to continue their work, and the base or carrier oils to moisturise and nourish the skin. Don't be surprised if the strokes in this treatment aren't particularly deep. They are simply designed to stimulate blood and lymph flow. The oils do the deep work and carry on working for some time after the treatment is over. They can relax muscle tension and work the tissue just as well as a Swedish massage can, but in a different way.

Treatments can vary greatly in cost, depending on where you go and where you are in the country. Do some research and try to get a practitioner through the personal recommendation of someone you know. Give yourself plenty of time and try to book a session during a period when you can rest directly after, or go home for some further relaxation.

Aromatherapy self massage

This is a similar way to use essential oils but not quite as wonderful as you have to do the work yourself! A self-massage sequence is included on pages 207–210. You should make sure the room is warm and that you are in a comfortable position, then apply the oil and rub it into your body just as if you were applying a moisturiser. Rub it all over your body, then wrap up warm and let yourself 'cook' for at least an hour. Leave the oils on for as long as possible, but if you are using an invigorating blend to wake yourself up you should shower the residue off before dressing.

Bathing or showering with essential oils

For both bath and shower the following steps should be taken to ensure you get the best from your treatment. The aromatherapy bath or shower is not a time for washing. If you need to wash do this before your 'treatment'. You should aim to leave the bath or shower with a thin film of oil left on your body to achieve the best effect; if you use the oils and finish off by soaping yourself all over, you will not be getting the best from the oils.

For bathing with essential oils, make sure that the room is warm, close the windows, then run the bath. Don't have the water too hot as you will want to stay in it for around 15 minutes. Once the bath has run you can sprinkle the correct and appropriate blend on the surface of the water. Get into the bath, then inhale deeply the benefits of the essential oils. When the bath is complete you should gently pat yourself dry so as to let the skin absorb the oils and continue their work. Dress and relax, or dress for a day or night out.

When you are using essential oils while showering, you cannot have the oil continually poured over you; you should therefore choose your blend and then place 2 or 3 drops on to a hot flannel. Get into the shower and close the doors. Start the shower and wait until the water vapour begins to fill the cubicle. Rub the flannel over your body during the shower and inhale the vapours. Leave the shower, then dry your body just as described for bathing.

Sauna/steam

You can get the fabulous effect of essential oils in both sauna and steam rooms. You may need to check with the owners before introducing the oils, and also with any fellow sauna or steam users. In the steam room you will need to add 2 or 3 drops of essential oil to the steam water outside of the cabin. In the sauna you should mix 2 or 3 drops with a ladle of water and then pour this on to the hot stones. Simply sit back, relax your breathing and inhale the oils deeply.

Inhalations

If you cannot get to a sauna you can create your own private inhalation. Pour boiling water into a large bowl and add the oils. Cover your head in a towel or teacloth, lean over the bowl and inhale deeply.

Compresses

Choose your oil and then place just a drop on a handker-chief or piece of cotton. Hold it near to your nose and mouth and inhale. This is the method you should employ if you want to use the oils throughout the night. Put an old pillowcase over your pillow to protect your good linen, then place a drop of oil on the surface. You can then inhale the oil throughout the night.

What amounts should I be using?

You should follow quantity guidelines very closely. If you decide on an inhalation to really invigorate yourself and the instructions on the bottle say to use 2 or 3 drops, then stick to 2 or 3 drops. Don't decide that you need a lot of invigoration and pour 10 drops into the bowl; at best you may feel nausea and at worst you will get a really bad headache and the vapour may even be too strong for your facial skin. Use the recommended amounts – remember that you are dealing with high-potency drugs.

Professional massage

The practitioner will blend the chosen oils ready for use according to their training. You don't need to worry about the quantities used as long as your therapist is professionally qualified. Just relax and enjoy the treat-ment.

Self massage

You will need to make your own massage blend to use in your treatment. The general rule is 1 drop of essential oil to each millilitre of base or carrier oil, not exceeding 8 drops of oil for any one treatment. This is definitely enough. You will need about 10 to 15 ml of oil for your first massage, but may get through more due to 'beginner's technique'. This will mean that 8 drops of essential oil to 15 ml of base oil is a very safe amount to use but still extremely effective. Remember that lots of the oil will be on your hands, some will be spilled and some will be left over.

Bathing or showering

As for the massage blend, you should use no more than 8 drops per bath, but this time you can dilute the oil in either a tablespoon of carrier or base oil, or a tablespoon of alcohol or milk dispersant. This ensures that the entire dosage is dispersed throughout the water rather than being left in one globule in the centre of the bath.

Sauna or steam

You will have to check with the operator of the facility you want to use, but you should not need to use more than 2 or 3 drops per session in a cupful of water.

Inhalations

Use 3 or 4 drops of oil in a bowl of water.

Compresses

Use 1 or 2 drops of oil on a cotton handkerchief or piece of fabric.

Terminology

There is some general terminology that should help you when choosing how to use essential oils as part of your Stay Young Detox programme.

Essential oil

The single, pure essence, this is probably the strongest version of the oil that you will be able to buy from either an aromatherapy company or a high street store.

Blended oil

Alternatively, you are likely to buy a blended oil. This can be either a blend of pure essential oil (several oils together in one bottle) or a blend of essential oils that have also been mixed in a carrier or base oil.

Carrier oil or base oil

This can be a vegetable oil or sweet almond, sunflower or grapeseed oil. Oils such as jojoba, avocado, and Macadamia nut are also available, but are more specialist.

Dispersant

A product such as milk or alcohol that will break up the drops of oil to disperse them so that single drops do not come into contact with naked, unprotected skin. This method is most useful for bathing.

CRYSTALS AND CRYSTAL HEALING

Crystals have their own energy, or resonance. They can be measured for energy just as any object can. Their different energy levels, resonance and density can tune in with our own energy, resonance and vibration. Once this tuning in occurs, we can reach homeostastis, or true balance.

Crystals are valuable in regrowth, regeneration and even rebirth, and can aid in detoxification, cleansing and healing. They are therefore invaluable in the Stay Young Detox programme.

There are many ways of using crystals. They can be held, worn or placed on your body. You can make tinctures out of them to take, or you can simply choose one that grabs your attention and let it do its work.

Crystals have been used for thousands of years, for adornment, protection and healing. They come from the earth and are formed over millions of years. If we could hear them talk they would have amazing stories to tell and tremendous wisdom and knowledge. Crystals can be precious jewels: diamonds and rubies, sapphires and emeralds. They can also be semi-precious stones, such as opals, amethysts and jasper. Whatever they are, they all have a purpose and meaning in gem and crystal therapy.

We take it for granted that wedding and engagement rings usually include diamonds. In crystal therapy the diamond signifies loyalty, fidelity and the bond between man and woman. It is the hardest gem we know, formed through many thousands of years of extreme heat to become the pure crystal we are so familiar with. The diamond is steadfast and true – completely appropriate in a piece of jewellery used for the marriage ceremony. We may not think that we are aware of crystal therapy, but we do consider it normal practice to have diamonds in our engagement rings. We probably just think that because a diamond ring is expensive it denotes commitment!

Crystals can help every situation and every emotion. For the purpose of the Stay Young Detox we will concentrate on ourselves. Staying young comes with confidence, self-belief and self-worth. Detoxing comes with cleansing and clearing. It also involves aspects of regrowth and regeneration. Any crystal that fulfils any or all of these aspects will be discussed.

We can look at the crystals and then consider how we can include them in our life, how they can boost and enhance – and how they can make us stay young in body, mind and spirit.

Types of crystal

Amber

Amber brings wisdom and balance. It holds secrets of the Earth. You may even find small insects from many millions of years ago nestled in the gem of resin. Amber is healing and can help with tissue and cell regrowth, and to purge dis-ease from the body. It can banish negative thoughts and energy, and is also a kidney tonic.

Tiger's eye

This is one of my favourite-looking crystals and therefore one of my most helpful crystals. Tiger's eye is for protection and can help you draw on your own resources for success without draining you. It can balance your digestion. It also helps you to develop your own intuition and is reported to give great confidence.

Opal

The opal cleanses the blood and kidneys and keeps insulin levels balanced. It encourages spontaneity and creativity but keeps you emotionally stable. Opals are good as a passion tool.

Rose quartz

Rose quartz is a stone of love. Its pinkish hue is romantic and healing. It helps with self-love as well as love for others, and works on the heart both emotionally and physically. It encourages circulation and blood flow, and brings about healing. Just looking at rose quartz makes you feel a warm glow inside.

Fluorites, all types

Fluorites come in many forms. They protect and are grounding and centring. They help to release toxins from the body and assist with cell growth and muscle damage. They can also help with creativity and sexuality.

Agates, including blue agate

Agates are calming and cooling, grounding and harmonising. They boost confidence and equip us with the ability to move on. Blue agate brings about balance and strengthens the bones by speeding up the healing process.

Labradorite

This oddly named crystal is fabulous for aiding digestion and metabolism. It protects and recharges, and enables us to promote our own intuition and insight. It is also the duty of labradorite to recharge all other stones on the planet. It cancels negative energy and promotes positive energy.

Emerald

Green emeralds are grounding and balancing, both physically and emotionally. They are calming and restful. Emeralds can enhance muscle healing and promote heart health. They will never let you forget, for they are stones of memory.

Lapis lazuli

Lapis is good for stress. It balances and harmonises on a mind, body and spirit level. It promotes immunity and cleansing, and creativity and objectivity. It is an all-round balancer.

Quartz

Although this is one of the more common stones it should not be undervalued, for it is probably also one of the most powerful stones. It is used to cleanse and revitalise. It may be used to dissipate bad energy and to regulate good energy. Quartz is often used near computer screens to prevent harmful rays and static, so it has a very physical use. It is also great for stimulating immunity.

Citrine

Citrine is less common than some of the stones, but just as valuable. It is balancing and cleansing, and works on the digestive system and the circulation. It also enhances creativity and encourages motivation.

Tourmaline

This stone is very cleansing, and great for detoxification. It purifies and boosts immunity and is very rejuvenating. It is also very balancing and grounding, as are many of the other green gem stones.

Malachite

This is another fabulous green stone with amazing properties. It is 'the stone of transformation', according to the British Fossil Association. It can help in times of great or small change, allowing you to move forwards, leaving the past in the past. It also helps with healing and cell growth, and with regeneration.

Sodalite

Sodalite is great for elimination. It boosts the kidneys and liver, and the metabolism and immunity. It is calming and balancing.

Amethyst

Like quartz, amethyst is a great all-rounder. It heals and protects. It helps the kidneys and liver, boosts circulation, balances the nervous system, boosts immunity, improves digestion and promotes heart health. Energetically, it cleanses auric fields and stimulates chakras. It is used in meditation and visualisation, and can often be found in a large crystal emanating energy and warmth.

Snowflake obsidian or Apache tears

This beautifully named crystal is a key stone for staying young. It encourages self-love and banishes self-doubt. It keeps balance through times of change, and allows you to move forwards while letting go of past fears or memories. It is a very positive stone, which keeps you in control when you most need to be in control. Snowflake obsidian also has beneficial skin-healing properties.

Turquoise

This Native American stone is most helpful with healing and protection. It promotes self-worth and self-realisation, and is supportive through change. Turquoise banishes negativity and promotes positive feelings of health and wealth. It is an all-round healer of the whole body, mind and spirit.

Using crystals

The above crystals are just a small selection of the more common stones, gems and crystals that we can use in crystal therapy, but they may just be enough to show you how they can support and enhance our lives. Crystals can be very personal, just as animal medicine is. Carrying crystals or wearing them can go totally unnoticed while getting us through some of life's stickier moments. If you don't want them with you during the day or evening, you can work with them in the privacy of your own home and then benefit from them while you go about your normal day.

You can approach crystal healing in many ways, but the two most useful are either to work out what you want help with, for example confidence, letting go, self-worth, cleansing and/or detoxing. You can then research which stones are the most appropriate and have them in jewellery, in their raw stone state or in polished or faceted pieces.

Alternatively, you can take yourself off to a gem or crystal shop, or fair, and choose something that catches your eye. Whatever its properties, it will be valuable to you and will help and promote health and happiness. Look up what you have chosen and see what it is that you are in need of or you need help with. The energy of crystals and stones is so old that it knows better than you what is needed and what will help!

Trust your crystals to do the best by you. You could even combine crystal medicine with animal medicine and imagine, for example, your cat animal medicine wearing a ruby crystal medicine collar. The combination is wonderfully powerful on a mind, body and spirit level. The visual image is very positive and pleasing, too.

YOGA

Yoga is the physical version of meditation. You could do yoga sessions at the start of each day of the 18-day programme. If you have never experienced yoga, book into a class and see just how invigorating and reviving it can feel. Every part of your body is stretched and life is breathed into every last nook and cranny. Yoga is very thorough and gives you fabulous flexibility.

Central to yoga is the belief that you are moving prana, or life energy, around the body. If you practise yoga regularly you are aiming to bring as much prana as possible into your body for strength and vital life.

In yoga, you use your body to effect a change on your mind and body instead of simply your breathing. But be warned, yoga is not simply a form of exercise for stretch-

'n'-tone. Some of the advanced moves in yoga techniques look as though they are completely above and beyond the bounds of human flexibility, but they are really quite attainable if they are taught correctly and if you build up to them. However, attempting extreme yoga techniques without first learning the basics is like attempting long division before addition – it will come to you eventually but should be respected and practised regularly. Having a relaxed mind will enable your body to 'work out' the moves; attempting them without relaxation is likely to cause injury. You will find that after practising yoga for a while you will be able to feel emotional, physical and mental calm.

Yoga is physical and as such it tones and works out the body, but it also tones the internal systems, such as the respiratory, circulatory and lymph systems. In addition, it works on the internal organs as some of the positions exert or release pressure in the organs and their surrounding areas. It stretches the muscles and keeps the joints supple and the spine healthy, supportive and strong.

Each yoga position holds a special purpose and usually has a name. A yoga sequence or session works all aspects of the body and frees everything up, so that mental and physical clarity are achieved. Breathing into the moves and holding them requires concentration and balance. However, there is nothing quick or sharp about yoga, and actually getting the body into some of the positions safely requires a process of gentle stretches, holding and concentration, which means that the focus has to be totally on your own mind and body, and nothing else can be considered.

As in the case of meditation, you should always start by attending a class or having lessons with a qualified and experienced yoga teacher. The yoga class will consist of relaxation and warming up exercises followed by a series of positions that may take some time to achieve. These will be interspersed with further relaxation and balancing before a further position is attempted. You are likely to need blankets, pillows, pads and layers of clothes, because the class will go from still and meditative, through physical, and back to stretching and relaxation. Always check what is required when you register with a class, and make sure the teacher knows your level. Teachers can work to all requirements, but enrolling in an advanced class to begin with will prevent you from getting the best out of it.

CHAKRAS

There are many chakras, but most people talk of seven or twelve. The main ones that you are likely to come across are those of the:

- Crown
- Third eye
- Throat
- Higher heart
- Heart
- Solar plexus
- Sacral
- Root

Each chakra is a source of energy related to its location on the body. Each chakra is a spinning wheel or disc – the word chakra means wheel. In yoga and Indian medicine, it is the balance and spinning of these wheels that tells us if we are in harmony and well. If any chakra is out of balance, this will mean disharmony and dis-ease.

Any practice that can bring the spinning back into rhythm or balance is beneficial. Many practitioners have been trained to open and spin the chakras and then to close them down to protect the person. This opening and closing is more a spinning into rhythm rather than a physical process. The work is done by passing intent or energy from one person to another so that harmony is achieved.

Moving our own energy, or chi

It may sound strange but we can work our own chi to get the best benefit. You have probably heard of people who talk about healing themselves by concentrating on sending good, healthy messages to a part of their body that is ill. By eating the right foods and doing the right exercises they can say they have healed themselves.

This can be hard to believe, but we can help ourselves to get better. It is no different than keeping a positive mind that releases positive energy and good endorphins into the body, rather than feeling bad or ill and losing the will to get better. This is not to say that anyone who becomes ill and doesn't recover simply doesn't want to get better (I am in no doubt that they do), but it is to say that you have a better chance of recovery if you feed your body with good food and positive thought and energy.

In order to get support from our own energy wheels we

can visualise their actions. You can call upon whatever strength or empowerment you need during your 18-day programme through your chakras.

Each chakra relates to an emotion or physical state or colour, among other things. The table below describes the associations and functions of each chakra in really basic terms. Read it and when you know what you need we can look at activating that property.

Chakra	Associated colour	Associated strength	Associated part of the body
Crown	Purple, gold and white	Spirituality	Top of head, top of skull
Third eye	Dark blue	Intuition and vision	Eyes
Throat	Lighter blue	Communication and self-expression	Mouth and throat
Higher heart	Green	Higher love of self	Heart
Heart	Green and pink	Love and relationships	Chest and lungs, circulation
Solar plexus	Yellow	Personal power and emotion, willpower	Digestion
Sacral	Orange	Emotional balance and sexuality	Genitalia, bladder, womb
Root	Red	Physical and base needs	Skeleton and bones

To capture chakra energy from your chosen chakra(s):

- Visualise the colour or a body part associated with the chakra(s) or the chakra(s) itself.

- Imagine a spinning wheel and try to speed it up or slow it down.

- Imagine the strength of colour and try to fade it or make it more vibrant.

- Imagine the body part and see it healthy and working, or slow it down to resting.

EXERCISE Example of how to use chakras

Imagine that you are going to have a busy day. You will be meeting with many friends; one of them is an old partner to whom you have not spoken for several years. As part of your Stay Young Detox you have decided to make conversation and bury old feelings once and for all – in other words, to make peace.

OK, you will need the throat chakra to be able to say what you truly mean. You will need the higher heart chakra to be true to yourself, and you will need the solar plexus chakra to stay calm and in control.

You don't need to lie down and meditate on this, and you don't need to do anything except in your own head unless you want to. Meditation is good but not entirely necessary.

Picture in your mind the throat, or the lighter blue, or your ability to express yourself. Whichever you visualise you can either activate or relax.

Imagine the light blue pulsing and relaxing your throat so that it is spinning easily and enabling you to say what you truly mean. Spin the wheel of the throat chakra energy and feel the support and openness it gives you. You are free to say what you feel.

Imagine the higher heart spot above your breast bone and just below your collar bone, and see the green colour. Visualise the green showing you that you are content with yourself. Your own higher love is peaceful and relaxed. You will feel the confidence you have that what you are doing is right. Your own self-belief will give you the confidence that you are on the right path. Spin the colour and feel it spread throughout your body. Be totally calm and self-aware.

Finally you can visualise the solar plexus. Feel the spot beneath your ribcage and above your stomach. See the yellow glow. See the warmth of the sun shining down on this spot and feeding you with your own personal power.

You can do anything you want to. You are positively glowing – quite literally, positively spinning and glowing. Now is the time to do what you need to do.

Once you have called upon your powers you need to put them away and protect yourself and them. If you leave them open they will leave you vulnerable and open to other people's energy. You need to conserve your own powers for your own personal use. Simply imagine all these points and chakras you have used. Imagine them slowing down and finally stopping in complete balance and harmony. They will still have their colours and their powers, but they will not have been activated for use.

They will just be waiting in the wings for the next time you want to use them.

Conversely, you may need to calm a chakra down during your Stay Young Detox. If you are frustrated or excited about something or if you are having doubts, you can complete the programme, then just check in with your body. How do you feel? What feels upset or out of balance?

Choose the most appropriate chakra or chakras – maybe the third eye is too open, or maybe you are imagining all sorts of things that won't actually be a problem. Your imagination and intuition are working overtime. Just see the colour or the body part and slow the spinning down. See it come calmly to a close and safely balanced.

Working with your own personal chakras gives you the power to help yourself in almost any situation. Calming and balancing, invigorating and exciting – you can choose.

SPACE CLEARING

Once you have decided to inject some vitality into your life on the Stay Young Detox, you may decide to inject the same energy into your home. Spring clean your space and then 'clear' it. Space clearing is the art of cleansing and consecrating buildings and homes. If you are looking to keep fresh and youthful in outlook, then it will be a perfect complement to rid yourself of old clutter or indeed anything that can stop you from moving forwards.

Space clearing involves the physical removal of rubbish, dirt and clutter, such as old magazines and newspapers lying around; old clothes that you no longer wear; foods that are past their sell-by date; crockery you don't use; old saucepans that have been replaced by newer, cleaner ones; make-up that you never wear; medicines that you should have thrown away for safety's sake; old bubble baths that you got for Christmas but never used; and the contents of several years of Christmas crackers that you cannot bear to throw away.

The spiritual removal of stale, stagnant, negative energy, or actual removal or recognition of energetic entities (ghosts), is perhaps more important than the removal of physical objects. It could include rooms you don't use; photo albums you have never sorted; thoughts to loved ones that have never been expressed; apologies that have gone unheard; confessions not made; arguments left unsettled; and old residents who have not left.

For the purposes of the Stay Young Detox we are going to look at simple space clearing techniques that you can start to introduce at home. There are many practitioners who would be more than happy to come to your home or office and space clear for you, but it might be good to start by seeing just what sort of difference you can make by introducing a few simple techniques.

At its most elementary, space clearing is just like physical spring cleaning. On a more detailed level it is about actually cleaning the energy of your home and thus making it like new, fully active, vibrant and full of energy.

Start by realising that you will not be able to take on the whole house overnight! Clearing will be a process that should be done thoroughly and systematically over the 18 days of the programme.

Choose a room that you spend most time in and you

will feel the benefits of your clearing much more immediately. Once you have chosen the room – for instance the living room – start clearing it out. It will be easy to see all the items that can be discarded almost immediately: rubbish, out-of-date magazines, old wrappers, the contents of the rubbish bin, and so on. There is nothing scientific about throwing away all the rubbish. The next step is to look at all the items in the room and decide if you really need or want them there. This is not to say that you should leave your room as empty as possible. You may like a lot of furniture. You just need to make sure that you are left with only useful, practical or beautiful items.

Once the room is clear of waste you need to set about actually physically cleaning it. Vacuum the whole room, move all the furniture and vacuum behind everything. Clean away the stale dust that has settled behind the sofa or taken up residence behind the Rembrandt! Polish every surface and wipe all the windows. Clean the telephone receiver and remove any dead leaves or flowers from house plants. Check down the sides of the chairs for crumbs or coins, and shake up the cushions so they are 'plump'. Generally ensure that the room is exactly how you would want it to be if you were arriving home after a long, hard day, ready to make you feel welcome and relaxed. You can then go on to clear every room in your house in the same way.

The following ideas show how to thoroughly space clear one room, and they apply to any room.

Bear in mind that space clearing will not be understood by everyone, so if you decide to space clear your own home you should choose to do it alone, when everyone else is out. To encourage the flow and cleansing of energy within your home, you should nurture it. We talk to pets and friends, and we also speak to the plants. Now it is time to talk to your home.

You should be clean and 'cleansed' yourself. Don't attempt space clearing in restrictive clothing; wear loose, comfortable clothes and relax into your task. You need to be receptive to the 'vibe' you get back from your rooms.

You can use chimes and bells during the course of clearing space, and can also utilise aromatherapy essential oils (*see page 152*) and flowers and petals. If the weather is fine, open the windows and let the air flow. Encourage energy to circulate by using incense or candles.

Scatter petals or spray essential oils in a water solution lightly around the room. Use a chime to sound in the darkest corners and highest points, and move the energy around every nook and cranny. Light candles to draw the air and circulate the atmosphere.

Wander around the room and feel each and every part of it; identify areas that feel colder and flatter and areas that feel energetic and active. Go around clapping loudly into each and every area to chase out the stagnant energy, and move the active energy around. Clap low and high.

Before you finish but after you have worked around every point of the room and energised every angle, walk around the perimeter of the room and stroke the energy in, encouraging forwards motion – as if you are encouraging something to pass you by. Once you have done this, the energy should be evenly distributed, cleansed and refreshed.

When you have finished, clear away your cleansing

equipment and then see how the room feels and how you feel along what you have just achieved. You now totally

PART **4**

Practical Section

10

Detox Recipes and Eating Suggestions

A balanced diet is essential for the detox programme to work well. It is the foundation upon which everything else rests.

It is often said that we should 'breakfast like kings, lunch like queens and supper like paupers'. I am not sure who first said this but it does have some truth. If we eat early in the day then we are up and about to use the energy the food produces. If we feast at midnight the body only has to sleep, so less energy is used up in activity.

In fact, the best way to nourish our bodies is to have 5 smaller meals a day rather than 3 or even 2 larger ones, which will make us swing between feeling very hungry and feeling very full. Having 5 smaller meals a day will make us feel constantly satisfied and will ensure that our bodies tick over very efficiently.

The recipes given here are made up entirely of super-foods – they are 'purist superfood'. Unless stated, all recipes are for one.

BREAKFASTS

MUESLI

1 small pot sheep's yoghurt
1 teaspoon sunflower seeds
1 teaspoon sesame seeds
1 teaspoon pumpkin seeds
1 dessertspoon blueberries or blackberries

Put the yoghurt in a bowl. Add the seeds and fruit. If you like runny yoghurt just add more. If you like your muesli to have a thick, paste-like consistency, one pot of yoghurt should be enough.

GRILLED GRAPEFRUIT AND HONEY

$1/2$ a grapefruit
1 teaspoon honey
1 tablespoon goat's yoghurt (optional)

Place the grapefruit on a baking tray or ovenproof dish. Smooth the honey over the top and place under a hot grill. When the honey has caramelised, remove it from the grill. Serve with the yoghurt if desired.

FRUIT SALAD

Mixture of your favourite fruits, such as blueberries, cherries and cranberries, either dried or fresh, or a combination – enough to fill a dessert bowl.
Juice of 1 fresh lime
1 dessertspoon honey

Mix the lime juice with the honey to a runny syrup. Pour the honey blend over the fruits. Stir gently until the fruits and juices are coated in the syrup.

SNACKS

The following are some ideas for small meals or snacks consisting totally of superfoods. There will be times on the detox programme when you will be unable to sit down to a main meal, or when you will just need something quick to eat to keep you going. You shouldn't get too hungry during the day if you eat five smaller meals rather than three larger ones as suggested; however, we are all human and the need to snack is a great one! There are many 'packet' snacks that you can carry around with you or have on stand-by as emergency measures. Choose any of the following to fill the gap and stop you from grabbing something to eat that is not totally detox.

Rice cakes

Make sure you buy the unsalted, and/or organic versions. You can get mini rice cakes or thin ones as an alternative to the more traditional thick slices.

Nuts and seeds

Incredibly high in antioxidants, nuts and seeds are ideal for on-the-move snacking. Don't eat too many as they are quite high in fat. They are, however, full of flavour and nutrients.

Pots of yoghurt

Mid-morning or mid-afternoon, a good way to fill up on healthy food is to have a pot of natural sheep's or goat's yoghurt. If you wish to enhance the flavour and add even more nutrition stir in a teaspoon of honey of your choice.

Crunchy vegetables

There is nothing to stop your chopping up some vegetables and taking them to work (or elsewhere outside your home) in your bag. Better still, don't bother with chopping – carrots are excellent for crunching whole – just discard the tops, unless your name is Bugs Bunny.

LIGHT MEALS

For something a little more substantial these light meals are some great ideas to get you started. You can prepare them in advance to take with you, and they can be made up in just a few minutes.

RED RICE SALAD

2 large tablespoons uncooked red rice

1 medium red onion, chopped or diced

Olive oil

Black pepper

1 fresh lime

1 tablespoon crumbled feta cheese

2 or 3 sprigs fresh coriander, finely chopped

Cook the rice following the instructions on the packet. Put a teaspoon of olive oil into a frying pan and fry the onion until slightly soft and browned at the edges. Add the cooked rice to the onion and stir so that the flavour of the onion in the oil is absorbed into the rice. Add 3 or 4 grinds of black pepper, then squeeze the lime juice into the pan. Transfer the rice and onions to a plate and scatter the cheese and coriander over the top. Pour the lime juice over the dish and serve.

GREEK SALAD

2 tablespoons cooked short-grain brown rice
1 50–100 g (2–4 oz) chunk of feta cheese, cubed – check that it is
    made from sheep's not cow's milk
1/2 a red onion, diced into small cubes
Black olives – approximately 6, but you can add more if desired
Handful watercress, finely chopped
Finely chopped fresh basil
Sesame oil
Lime juice

Put the rice on a plate and place the cheese on top, then scatter the onions and the olives over the rice. Scatter the watercress and basil over the top. Mix the ingredients together. Blend the sesame oil and the lime juice and use as a dressing for the salad.

ROAST BROCCOLI WITH TUNA

1 tablespoon brown rice
Olive oil
1 large flower broccoli, split into florets
1 fillet cooked fresh tuna, flaked
1 teaspoon toasted/shredded almonds
Juice of 1 lime
1 tablespoon coriander, finely chopped
Black pepper

Boil the rice according to the instruction on the packet. While it is cooking, heat a roasting tray containing a tablespoon of olive oil in the oven. When the oil is hot place the broccoli florets on the tray, roast for 5 minutes, then turn and continue to roast until they are slightly browned and soft in the middle. When the rice is cooked, mix it with the flaked tuna and the almonds. Toss with the lime juice, a teaspoon of olive oil and coriander, and place on a dinner plate. When the broccoli is done place it on the bed of rice and tuna. Serve with a twist of fresh black pepper.

YOGHURT DIPS

Any of the vegetables from the list of superfoods – enough to
    fill a serving plate
1 pot sheep's yoghurt
Juice of 1 lemon
Handful watercress and coriander, finely chopped
1 small onion, finely diced
1 clove of garlic, finely diced
Rice cakes – enough for a lunchtime snack

Chop the vegetables into bite-sized crudités. Mix the yoghurt with the lemon juice, herbs, onion and garlic, and place in a small serving bowl. Dip the vegetables and/or rice cakes into the yoghurt dip, and enjoy.

HOT GRILLED CABBAGE

$1/2$ a small cabbage – red is preferable
$1/2$ a red onion, finely chopped
1 tablespoon cooked wild rice
Soft goat's cheese
Cayenne pepper

Slice the red cabbage and stir-fry so that it is crunchy but not totally raw. You can alternatively steam or boil it – use whichever is your preferred method. Fry the onion until it is translucent but still crunchy, then add the cabbage and put in a serving bowl. Scatter the wild rice and break the soft cheese over the top. Season lightly with the cayenne pepper. Grill until the cheese is toasted on top but not burnt.

TUNA RICE

1 small can or medium fillet tuna
Olive oil
1 heaped tablespoon cooked rice
1 tablespoon red kidney beans, cooked or canned
2 small beetroot, cooked or pickled
Balsamic vinegar

Grill the tuna with olive oil. Flake the tuna and mix together with the rice and kidney beans. Dice the beetroot and sprinkle on top of the tuna, rice and bean mixture. Combine vinegar and olive oil to your taste to make a dressing. Pour 2 teaspoons of the dressing over the fish mixture.

NUT SALAD

2 tablespoons cashew nuts
2 tablespoons pine nuts
1 cooked beetroot, shredded or sliced
Watercress, shredded
2 tablespoons chopped coriander leaves
1 carrot, grated
4 tablespoons nut or olive oil
Juice of 1/2 a lemon
Poppy seeds

Toss all the ingredients together and serve. Alternatively, you can serve this dish on a bed of brown rice or as an accompaniment to any of the main course dishes in this section.

SARDINES AND DRIED CRANBERRIES

2 tablespoons short-grain brown rice
2 grilled fresh or canned sardines, boned and flaked
Small chunk soft goat's or sheep's cheese, cubed
Handful dried cranberries or cherries, or both, soaked for
   1 hour in water
Lime juice
Pistachio oil

Cook the rice according to the instructions on the packet. Place in a bowl and add the sardines. Mix together. Add the cheese and the soaked fruits and mix together. Dress with a blend of lime juice and pistachio oil to taste.

TOMATO GAZPACHO

4 large tomatoes, or 1 large can tomatoes, chopped

1 small cooked beetroot

2 fresh cloves of garlic

Juice of 1 lemon

Juice of 1 lime

1 tablespoon olive oil

Freshly ground black pepper

1 dessertspoon sheep's yoghurt

Place all the ingredients in a blender and blend until everything has been combined together and the colour of the mixture is red. You can blend the mixture further if you like smooth soups, or leave it chunky if you prefer. Chill the soup for at least an hour in the fridge, then serve in a bowl with the yoghurt lightly stirred into it.

GARLIC AND GINGER VEGETABLES WITH GOAT'S OR SHEEP'S CHEESE

Large portion mixed carrots, broccoli and shredded cabbage, either red or green

4 tablespoons water

1 teaspoon crushed ginger

2 cloves of fresh garlic, finely chopped

1 tablespoon hard goat's or sheep's cheese, grated

Small sprig of coriander, finely chopped

Chop the vegetables into narrow strips. Place in a large dish and mix in the water, ginger and garlic. Strew the cheese over the top. Bake slowly in a preheated 180°C/350°F/Gas 4 oven for about 50 minutes, or until the vegetables are tender. Serve with more fresh ginger and coriander scattered over the top.

BEETROOT AND FETA MELT

2 medium-sized beetroots
1 tablespoon olive or nut oil
$1/2$ a teaspoon honey
Juice of 1 lemon
Handful watercress stems
1 tablespoon feta cheese, cubed
1 tablespoon roasted pine kernels

Peel and wash the beetroots, then roast them in a preheated 180°C/350°F/Gas 4 oven for half an hour, or until tender. Cut into quarters. Mix together the oil, honey and lemon juice. Place the watercress on a dinner plate, and arrange the beetroot quarters on top. Scatter the cheese and pine kernels over the top. Combine the olive oil, honey and lemon, and drizzle over the dish.

GARLIC STARTER

This kind of starter is served in many restaurants but using crusty bread rather than rice cakes.

1 medium-sized bulb of garlic
4 or 5 large rice cakes or 10 cocktail-sized cakes
Olive oil, for dipping
Lemon juice, to taste

Roast the garlic in a preheated 200°C/400°F/Gas 6 oven for 30 minutes. Check that it is cooked through by seeing if the individual cloves are soft if you squeeze them. Serve the garlic bulb on a small side plate and simply squeeze the contents of each clove on to a rice cake. Spread the garlic over the cake and crunch away. For extra nutrients you can drizzle on a little olive oil and a squeeze of lemon juice.

MAIN COURSES

OVEN-BAKED STUFFED TOMATOES

1 large tomato
Creamed or soft goat's cheese
Basil leaves, chopped
1 clove of garlic, finely sliced
Cooked brown rice
Cooked black beans
Olive oil
Sesame seeds, normal or ready toasted

Hollow out the tomato and place on a baking tray in a preheated 180°C/350°F/Gas 4 oven for 10 minutes to soften. Lightly stir-fry the goat's cheese, basil leaves, garlic, brown rice and beans. Stuff the tomato with this mixture and drizzle with some olive oil. Bake for a further 10 minutes, or until piping hot. Scatter sesame seeds over the top to taste and serve.

SALMON AND TARRAGON

1 fillet salmon

Handful watercress on stems

1 dessertspoon tarragon leaves, chopped

2 tablespoons cooked brown rice

1 teaspoon honey

1 teaspoon sunflower oil

Juice of 1 lime

Grill the salmon fillet until pink and tender. Chop together the watercress and tarragon and mix into the brown rice. Put the honey, oil and lime juice in a cup and stir together, or shake together in a jar. Put the rice on a serving plate, place the salmon fillet on top and pour the dressing over the top.

NUTTY MACKEREL

Spring onions, sliced

10 cloves of garlic

Cayenne pepper

3 tablespoons walnut oil

1 piece smoked mackerel, flaked

1 large tomato or several small cherry tomatoes, chopped

2 tablespoons crushed walnuts

300 ml (1/2 pint) vegetable stock

Parsley, finely chopped

Squeeze of lemon juice

Fry the onions, garlic and cayenne pepper in the walnut oil until the onions are translucent. Add the fish flakes and tomato and fry for 5 minutes. Add the walnuts and stock and fry for a further 5 minutes. Serve with the chopped parsley and a squeeze of lemon juice.

RED ONION AND SALMON CEVICHE

This recipe requires very fresh salmon but is superb, simple, very healthy and wonderful for entertaining.

1 fresh salmon fillet
Juice of 2 fresh limes
1 medium-sized red onion
1/4 of a fennel bulb
1 sprig dill
Oil, to drizzle

Cut the salmon into thin strips and marinade in the lime juice for at least 2 hours; make sure that the fish is covered with the juice. Slice the onion into very thin strips or very thin hoops. Cut the fennel into equally thin slices.

You will know that the fish is ready when it has turned opaque. Place the fish strips on a plate and scatter the onion and fennel over the top. Garnish with the dill and drizzle oil over the top to taste.

HERB AND VEGETABLE LAYERS

2 large tomatoes, sliced
1/4 of a cabbage, shredded
1 slice goat's/sheep's cheese roulade, approximately 1 cm
  (1/2 in) thick
1 slice white onion, approximately 1 cm (1/2 in) thick
1 sprig fresh oregano
1 sprig fresh rosemary

Grill the tomatoes until brown, then set aside. Stir-fry the cabbage quickly in a hot pan or wok until slightly browned but still crisp and green, then set aside. Place the onion slice in a hot, non-stick pan, and fry in a trace of oil until it is golden but not falling apart. Turn over to make sure both sides are cooked through. While the onion is frying, place the oregano and rosemary in the corner of the pan to heat. Remove from the heat. When the herbs have cooled, crush the stalks so that the leaves fall off onto a plate. Discard the stalks.

Place some tomato slices on an ovenproof plate. Scatter some of the herbs over the top, then place the onion slice on top. Put the cheese roulade and the remaining tomatoes on the onion slice. Top with the remaining herbs and put the plate in a preheated 220°C/425°F/Gas 7 oven for just long enough for the cheese to melt a little at the edges and begin to drip down. Serve on a bed of shredded cabbage.

BEANS AND HERBS

5 or 6 spring onions, topped, tailed and split down the middle
  at the green end
Large handful fresh broad beans
2 or 3 broccoli florets
¼ of a fennel bulb, finely chopped
Sprigs of dill, parsley and coriander
Sunflower oil
Juice of 1 lemon
Freshly ground black pepper
Soft sheep's cheese

Drop the spring onions into a bowl of iced water – the ends should curl if the water is cold enough; remove from the water once they have curled over. Mix together the beans, spring onions, broccoli and fennel. Put on a plate. Chop the herbs or rip the leaves and sprinkle over the bean mix. Drizzle the oil over the salad to taste, then squeeze the lemon onto the plate through your hands, so that the pips stay off the plate. Season with black pepper and crumble the cheese over the top. You can either serve this dish cool and fresh, or place the plate under the grill for a couple of minutes, until the cheese begins to brown and melt.

BROCCOLI AND ALMOND RISOTTO

3 tablespoons olive oil

100 g (4 oz) small onions

4 or 5 broccoli florets, sliced into small pieces

4 cups vegetable stock

1 clove of garlic, chopped

2 cups uncooked brown rice

100 g (4 oz) grated pecorino romano cheese

Large handful toasted shredded almonds

Chopped coriander, to garnish

Heat the olive oil and fry the onions until they are translucent. Put the broccoli florets in a pan. Add the onions and the oil, together with a cup of stock, and cook over a medium heat for 5 minutes. Add the chopped garlic, the rest of the stock and the rice, and simmer until the rice has absorbed all the liquid. Stir in the cheese and wait for it to look as if it is just beginning to melt. Serve in a large bowl with the almonds and the coriander scattered over the top.

DESSERTS

Just because you are detoxing it doesn't mean that you cannot have healthy helpings of pudding – *desserts* are the reverse of *stressed* after all!

SUMMER FRUIT COMPOTE

Mixture of berries, such as blackberries, raspberries, strawberries
   and blueberries
Natural honey
Sheep's yoghurt
Toasted sesame seeds

Gently simmer together the fruits and a tablespoon of
honey until the fruits are soft. Place the mixture in a bowl
and top with a tablespoon of the yoghurt mixed with a
teaspoon of honey. Scatter the toasted sesame seeds over
the top and serve.

CHERRY SOUP

1 pot of yoghurt
10–15 cherries, stoned and crushed
1 teaspoon honey
A few mint leaves, to decorate

Mix or blend the yoghurt together with the cherries and
honey. Pour into a dessert bowl and decorate with the
mint leaves.

FRUIT CRUMBLE

Mixture of cherries, berries and other fruits from the list of
   superfoods – enough to totally fill a dessert bowl
2 teaspoons honey
1/2 a teaspoon fresh grated ginger
Mixture of nuts and seeds of your choice – enough for 2 large
   tablespoons

Put the fruits and honey in a pan and heat gently until the fruits are softened but not mushy, then stir in the ginger. Crush the nuts and seeds in a pestle and mortar, or place in a plastic bag and crush with a rolling pin or bottle. Put the fruits in a bowl and cover with the nut crumble. Bake for 20 minutes in a preheated 200°C/400°F/Gas 6 oven, or grill until the crust is golden brown.

11

Body Care Manual

Thermotherapy showers, dry skin brushing, drinking at least 1.5 litres (3 pints) of water a day and exfoliation are crucial to any detoxification programme. They may seem old hat and unoriginal but there is nothing old hat in the fact that they work, and that they speed up the detox process beyond measure. Without them, you would really need to add another few weeks to your programme! Do them and feel the effects almost immediately.

THERMOTHERAPY SHOWERING OR BATHING

There is nothing new in taking a cold shower to refresh and invigorate yourself. In Nordic countries, people may go straight from a sauna into snow, and in some places people have wooden buckets of ice-cold water poured over them for the short, sharp shock treatment. What is new is our understanding of exactly what this alternation of extreme temperatures can do to the body – the theory behind thermotherapy.

As soon as our body is subjected to warmth for a short period of time, the following chemical changes occur within it:

- **Vasodilation**   A widening of the blood vessels, increasing blood supply throughout the body.

- **Increased circulation**   The vasodilation floods the body with oxygenated blood.

- **Increased metabolism**   Improves the rate at which the body processes foods and toxins, and burns energy.

- **Increased pulse rate**   Increases circulation and pumps the heart faster.

- **Increased cell metabolism**   The rate at which the body manufactures good chemicals, e.g. hormones, is improved.

- **Increased lymph function**   Improves the body's ability to clean waste materials and expel them from the body; the body's waste-disposal system is accelerated.

The simple process of heating up the body makes it deeply relaxed, and bodily functions take place more efficiently. All these functions increase and promote the body's ability to clean and regenerate itself, and to function at an optimum level.

These effects occur after 4 or 5 minutes' exposure to deep warmth. We know exactly how we feel when we walk into a warm, cosy room; we relax, feel good and breathe more easily. However, if we stay in that warm room or under that warm duvet and become too warm we need to cool down. If we don't and the heat keeps on coming, we begin to feel claustrophobic, or as if we are cooking or simply very uncomfortable, and then everything really slows down as our bodies try to cope with the excess heat. It is like being in a sauna or steam room and feeling really good, and then just a short time later feeling that you need to get out because the heat has become unbearable. That is exactly what happens if you are exposed to heat for too long.

With correctly applied thermotherapy treatments, this is when the cold is introduced. The application of cold in the short term, that is 2 or 3 minutes, has the following effects:

- **Vasoconstriction** The narrowing of blood vessels restricting blood supply to areas, pulling blood from the surface to the core of our body.

- **Analgesic effect** The release by the body of a natural pain relief substance (prostaglandin), which in turn relaxes the muscles. This is often described as numbing, but is in fact the sensation of natural pain relief.

- **'Shock' effect of temperature change** The circulation/oxygenation of the blood is increased.

- **The release of necrosin is inhibited** This natural chemical, which destroys tissue, stops being released into the body, so that damage to the muscles is prevented.

The application of cold immediately makes the body more comfortable after the heat. The circulation continues to increase, and the flow of blood through the muscles keeps them toned and honed.

Of course, you couldn't stand under a cold shower for too long – long-term exposure to the cold is dangerous. The body slows to a stop to protect our core functions, and hypothermia sets in.

A correctly applied thermotherapy treatment involves the alternate use of hot and cold over a period of time to continually benefit from the excellent effects of hot and cold on the body.

There can be no doubt that increased blood flow throughout the body; a reduction in muscle damage; fully oxygenated, fully circulating blood; an efficiently pumping heart; and the continuous toning of skin and muscles is just the kind of thing that can enhance the Stay Young Detox programme.

So, take a shower and swap the temperature from cold to hot at least 3 times for at least 30 seconds each time. Do this every day and I promise you it will feel absolutely great. Your skin will glow and your body will be fighting fit. It truly is that simple.

If you don't shower run a bath of hot water, take a plastic jug into the bath with you and, just before finishing the bath, pour a jug of ice-cold water over your head and shoulders. Slip down and immerse yourself in the hot water, then repeat with the cold water. Do this 3 times and you have experienced thermotherapy.

SELF MASSAGE

There is no science to self-massage techniques. We probably massage ourselves every day in a great way without even being aware of it. However you massage yourself, it will have a brilliant effect on the body and skin. Also remember that when you carry out self massage you benefit not only from the massage effects, but also from the action of actually doing the massage – something you don't get when paying for a professional treatment.

As is the case with thermotherapy, massage can increase blood flow, warm the body so that its ability to absorb oils such as essential oils is increased, and relax and tone the muscles. It can make the body release good hormones such as seratonin – a feel-good chemical. It can also increase the efficiency of the lymph system, which will help in the internal cleansing of waste products and toxins.

The actual carrying out of a massage helps to develop muscle tone, increases blood supply further due to the 'exercise' you are doing, and moisturises your hands and body with the base or carrier oil.

Rather than thinking of particular massage strokes or techniques you should think of all the things you can do that can already be called massage:

- **Soaping your body in the bath**   You rub your body in firm, circular movements all over.

- **Drying off with a towel**   You use the towel to make sure that every part of your body is dry; you cover the entire surface of your body, and you rub quite vigorously.

- **Moisturising your body**   You rub cream or gel all over your body, paying particular attention to specific areas of dryness.

- **Washing your hair**   You rub your scalp to make sure that the shampoo has reached the roots of your hair.

The movements consist of firm circles around the scalp and behind the ears.

- **You carry out your skin care routine**   This is similar to washing, but you pay particular attention to the more gentle or sensitive areas, using a different, more appropriate product.

There really is nothing to change except perhaps the time you take to carry out these processes and the temperature of the room.

Make sure that the room is warm. It is preferable to do self massage after you have just had a bath or shower, when your skin is most receptive, so you don't want to get cold. You should also allow at least 15 minutes for the massage – this should be relaxing and enjoyable.

Sit or stand in a comfortable position, then start the massage. Begin with the feet and work up to the head via the legs, knees, thighs, buttocks, stomach, arms and hands, elbows, torso, neck and face. Finish with a great scalp rub, just as if you were shampooing your hair. Don't worry about getting oil in your hair as it will moisturise and condition your scalp and the hair itself.

You may decide to mix a massage oil especially for the purpose of your self massage, or to choose a blend that is pre-prepared. I would recommend an anti-cellulite blend or cleansing blend simply because it is not only anti-cellulite but also very detoxifying. It will contain diuretic properties to prevent water retention and will be extremely balancing and uplifting – and it will smell good, too.

ANTI-CELLULITE RECIPE

2 tablespoons oil – sunflower, grapeseed, or even olive oil is good

2 drops juniper essential oil

2 drops lemon essential oil

2 drops rosemary essential oil

Combine the oils in a bowl. The juniper, lemon and rosemary oils have extremely detoxifying, cleansing, stimulating and diuretic properties. The base oil enables the oils to work safely over the skin and moisturise at the same time.

When you have finished your massage, you should ideally wrap up warm and relax for at least an hour. If the purpose of the massage was to wake you up and invigorate you, carry out the treatment and then shower – remember the invigoration of the thermotherapy shower! – and then dry off, get dressed and paint the town red.

DRY SKIN BRUSHING

Dry skin brushing speeds up the lymph flow, the body's waste-disposal system, and sloughs away any dead skin cells on the surface of the body. If you carry out skin brushing every day you will feel the benefits in just 3 or 4 days. The skin will become soft and supple, and the circulation will be increased throughout the body.

Dry skin brushing is also great for treating cellulite, as it helps the body to excrete waste fluids and excess fluids. It speeds up the efficiency of fluid flow between tissue, and prevents or reduces the pooling of fluid or the retention of water. It does all this and it is extremely simple to do.

All you need is a bristle brush, linen mitt or dry flannel or towel. Just find something that has a mildly abrasive surface made of bristle or fabric.

Make sure that your skin is dry and that all the strokes you make flow upwards. Imagine that you are trying to paint your body from top to toe in big, sweeping brushstrokes towards your head. The strokes should be firm and rigorous, but slightly more gentle when working over the more delicate skin of the stomach and breasts, the backs of the knees, the armpits and the facial area.

EXFOLIATION

Exfoliation is the wet version of dry skin brushing. It sloughs off dead skin cells, leaving the skin soft and glowing.

There are hundreds of exfoliating products, both natural and synthetic, on the market. Keep them in the shower and exfoliate on a regular basis – every 2 days is ideal. Exfoliation of your face should be done less often, as you don't want to overstimulate the sebaceous glands.

Simply rub the exfoliant over your entire body in small circles, using firm strokes. Pay particular attention to areas of dry skin, on the elbows, knees and soles of your feet. Once the exfoliation is complete you should step into a warm shower or bath and continue rubbing until all the scrub has been washed away.

Here are some home-grown exfoliating scrubs to try.

RICE POLISH

3 large tablespoons white rice (this is the only time white refined rice is appropriate on any detox programme!)

1 pot natural yoghurt – this can be normal dairy yoghurt

2 or 3 drops eucalyptus essential oil

Grind the rice in a blender or coffee grinder; alternatively, break down the grains in a pestle and mortar. Do not grind them too finely, as they should still be quite coarse. Mix the ground rice into a paste with the essential oil.

Massage the mixture all over your body, avoiding the eyes and any broken or sensitive areas of skin. When your entire body has been covered, wash off the mixture with firm strokes. Once the mixture has been washed away, smooth the yoghurt all over your body, leave for 5 minutes to moisturise and soften the skin, then rinse away.

HONEY BODY SMOOTHER

2 large tablespoons sesame seeds

2 large tablespoons base or carrier oil of your choice

2 tablespoons honey – clear not solid

2 drops lavender essential oil

Mix all the ingredients together in an ovenproof dish or pan. Heat the blend until warm, either on the hob or in the oven, or for just 15 seconds in the microwave. Check the temperature before using the blend.

Rub the mixture all over your body, again in firm, circular strokes. Leave the blend on your body for at least 5 minutes, but watch out that you don't get everything in your bathroom sticky! Wash off with warm water, then pat dry with a warm towel.

SIMPLE SALT SCRUB

2 tablespoons natural sea salt for a rough scrub, or refined salt for a
   more gentle scrub
2 tablespoons carrier oil
2 drops juniper essential oil
2 drops ginger essential oil

Mix all the ingredients together in a bowl, then use as a scrub to exfoliate the entire body. This warming, relaxing and diuretic blend will speed up the flow of excess fluids. Leave on for 5 to 10 minutes, then rinse off.

Magnesium bathing

The simplest way to get a concentration of magnesium is to use Epsom salts. These are readily available in most chemists or health food stores.

Run a hot bath, quite deep to get the best effect. Pour into the bath approximately 1 kg (2 lb) of Epsom salts, and stir until completely dissolved. Simply get into the bath and relax, breathing deeply through the nose and out through the mouth. Spend at least 10 minutes relaxing in the bath – do absolutely nothing except relax!

Slowly get out of the bath and dry yourself off. You will feel very warm and quite 'glowing'. This will not be solely from the effect of the bath but also from the magnesium that is drawing the toxins from your body.

You must continue to relax after the bath, so having the bath last thing at night and going off to bed is ideal. If you are going to bed wrap up warm and relax – read a book, watch a film or just snooze.

Relaxation sequence

Taking time to relax and let your body get on with the cleansing process is crucial to the successful completion of your detox programme. You should aim to find time to relax as often as possible during the programme (and also long after it). A little and often is far more effective than once in a blue moon.

Just as in 'power napping', if you carry out a meditation or relaxation exercise for only 10 minutes each day you should find yourself much more grounded, centred and in control.

EXERCISE Total relaxation

You can prepare a room specially for the purpose, or just take yourself to a quiet place in your head. Ignore all outside stimuli and concentrate on yourself; you are the most important part of your relaxation.

• Lie down on the floor, sit comfortably in a chair or just close your eyes.

• Start to breathe in deeply through your nose, then hold for a count of 4 and release for a count of 8.

• After breathing correctly for a couple of minutes you should find that your breathing has slowed down and feels very natural. You can stop counting.

• Now start to consider how your body is feeling. As you

inhale start thinking about your feet and the ankle areas of your body. Are they tense? If so, relax them.

- As you exhale, picture the air you breathe out to be the old, stagnant air, and the air you breathe in as new, fresh air.

- Think of your calves and knees. Picture the warm air travelling through any tense muscles, bathing them in light. Exhale the stale air.

- Picture your knee joints and your upper leg areas; breathe deeply and relax.

- Feel the air being breathed into the groin area, relaxing the tension and soothing the pelvis. Breathe out the bad air.

- See the golden light swirling around your stomach and abdomen, cleansing and uplifting your centre of emotion and spirit.

- Watch the light thread its way between each rib, filling the lungs and the chest cavity with warm, expanding air.

- Watch each of your fingers fill with golden light and spread through your fingers up your lower arms.

- Breathe the energy into your shoulders and the base of your neck. Feel your neck relax and melt into the floor and up into the base of your skull.

- The light may now travel into the root of each of your hair follicles, making your scalp feel invigorated and tingling.

- Each time you exhale you are breathing out waste, stress and anything you don't want in your life. Each time you breathe in you are breathing in new life, relaxation and contentment.

- Once you have renewed the life inside your body, you should look to see where the source of your new breath and new light is.

- Take yourself to a place that you have enjoyed – it could be by the seashore, in a country field or relaxing at home.

- See yourself in this place, watch yourself enjoying it and being content, and feel how it feels.

- Take time to remember what it feels like to be in such a wonderful place. Check in with your emotions to remember what it is like to be truly happy and relaxed.

- Take a mental picture of the scene you have chosen. Set this picture and your feelings in your mind, just like a snapshot of a total moment in time.

- When you are ready, start to think about bringing your consciousness back into your own body and into the room you are in.

- Open your eyes slowly, and if you are lying down roll over on to your side. Wait a few moments before you eventually push yourself up to sitting and then to standing.

You should feel totally relaxed, centred and grounded – get on with your day and with your Stay Young Detox. If anything at any stage gets to you or upsets you, simply recall the photo from your memory bank, and remember the feelings of calm.

EXERCISE Whole body sequence

- Walk up and down 10 steps or stairs for 5 minutes at a normal pace.

- Stand with your feet shoulder-width apart and alternately lift your left leg and left arm up and out to the side, then your right leg and right arm up and out to the side. Repeat 10 times on each side. Keep your arms and legs slightly bent while you carry out this step.

- Standing in the same position as before, clasp your hands in front of your nose with the arms slightly bent. Keeping your shoulders relaxed, twist slowly from side to side. The stretch will increase gradually and you should end it when you can see directly behind yourself. Feel the stretch in your stomach and waist muscles. Repeat 10 times on each side.

- Walk on the spot for 5 minutes, making sure that you bring each knee up to hip level. Swing your arms up and down in a marching motion, bringing your hands up to shoulder height.

- Walk on the spot for 5 minutes, bringing your knees up and out to the side to hip level. Clasp your hands in front of you with your forearms close together. As you step, lift your arms and lower them. Do not let your arms drop below shoulder height.

- Jog on the spot for 5 minutes without lifting your toes from the floor. Lift your heels up and down and wiggle your hips as much as possible.

- Facing forwards, twist your head slowly from side to side. Look over your right and left shoulder alternately. Hold the stretch for a moment and release, then look over your other shoulder.

- Standing with your feet shoulder-width apart, hold the back of an upright chair. Lower your body down until your knees are bent at 90 degrees, hold the position for the count of 5 and lift up slowly. Repeat 15 times. Remember to clench your buttocks and thighs as you lift and lower your body.

- Kneel on the floor with your hands shoulder-width apart, flat on the floor. Walk your hands forwards so that you are leaning your body weight on to your hands and using your knees as a balance. Keeping your back straight, bend and lower your arms until your nose touches the floor and then lift. Repeat 10 times, slowly.

Resources

These addresses are useful for finding out what you might need on your Stay Young Detox programme. Contact the appropriate organisation to obtain the names of fully qualified, registered practitioners in your area.

Organisations

British Complementary Medicine Association
9 Soar Lane
Leicester
LE3 5DE
0116 242 5406

Institute for Complementary Medicine
PO Box 194
London
SE16 1QZ
020 7237 5165

Aromatherapy Organisations Council
3 Latymer Close
Braybrooke
Market Harborough
LE16 8LN
01858 434242

British Acupuncture Council
Park House
206–208 Latimer Road
London
W10 6RE
020 8964 0222

Colonic International Association
16 Englands Lane
London
NW3 4TG
020 7483 1595

Association of Reflexologists
27 Old Gloucester Street
London
WC1 3XX
0990 673320

Transcendental Meditation
Freepost
London
SW1P 4YY
0990 143733

Yoga for Health Foundation
Ickwell Bury
Ickwell Green
Biggleswade
SG18 9EF

The School of Feng Shui
2 Cherry Orchard
Shipston on Stour
Warwickshire
CV36 4QR
01608 664998
info@fengshui-school.co.uk
www.fengshui-school.co.uk

Suppliers

The Edward Bach Centre
(Bach Flower Remedies)
Mount Vernon
Bakers Lane
Sotwell
Wallingford
OX10 0PZ
01235 550086

Aromatherapy Associates Ltd
(Aromatherapy blends)
PO Box 14981
London
SW6 2WH
020 7371 9878

Essential oils

Fleur Oils
0800 980 7600

Fragrant Earth
01458 831216

Further suggestions

Exfoliation, body brushing, depilation and moisturising products are all easily and generally available from supermarket chains, department stores and high street chemists.

Vitamin supplements are available from either health food stores or high street chemists. They are becoming increasingly available from supermarket chains. Make sure you try to get yeast-, wheat- and additive-free varieties.

Make-up is available from high street chemists and supermarkets, but you should also be able to get a free consultation from most department stores at one of their beauty counters. They normally hope you will buy enough products to pay for the consultation, but it should come free of charge!